CASES IN MEDICAL MICROBIOLOGY AND INFECTIOUS DISEASES

CASES IN MEDICAL MICROBIOLOGY AND INFECTIOUS DISEASES

Peter H. Gilligan, Ph.D.
Associate Director, Clinical Microbiology-Immunology
Laboratories, University of North Carolina Hospitals
Associate Professor, Departments of
Microbiology & Immunology and Pathology
University of North Carolina School of Medicine
Chapel Hill, North Carolina 27514

Daniel S. Shapiro, M.D.
Clinical Instructor in Medicine
Fellow in Clinical Microbiology and Infectious Diseases
University of North Carolina Hospitals
Chapel Hill, North Carolina 27514

M. Lynn Smiley, M.D.
Head, Clinical Virology Section
Burroughs-Wellcome Company
Research Triangle Park, North Carolina 27709
Clinical Associate Professor, Medicine (Infectious Diseases)
University of North Carolina School of Medicine
Chapel Hill, North Carolina 27514

American Society for Microbiology
Washington, DC

Library of Congress Cataloging-in-Publication Data

Gilligan, Peter H., 1951–
  Cases in medical microbiology and infectious diseases / by Peter
H. Gilligan, Daniel S. Shapiro, and M. Lynn Smiley.
    p.   cm.
  Includes index.
  ISBN 1-55581-045-4
  1. Medical microbiology—Case studies. I. Shapiro, Daniel S.,
1959–   . II. Smiley, M. Lynn, 1952–   . III. Title.
  [DNLM: 1. Communicable Diseases—microbiology—case studies.
2. Diagnosis, Differential—case studies. WC 100 G481c]
QR46.G493   1992
616.9—dc20
DNLM/DLC
for Library of Congress   92-10690
                                                                CIP

Dedicated to the memory of

Phillip J. Bassford, Jr., Ph.D.

whose belief and encouragement
helped bring this book
to reality

CONTENTS

INTRODUCTION

The goal of this text is simple yet ambitious. It is to challenge students to develop a working knowledge of the various disciplines of medical microbiology, including bacteriology, mycology, parasitology, and virology. We believe many students are more enthusiastic about learning information if they can see how it directly relates to patient care. By studying case histories of patients seen at a university teaching hospital, students will better understand the importance of mastering basic medical microbiology facts and concepts.

The cases are presented as "unknowns" and are accompanied by several questions designed to test knowledge in four broad areas:

(i)   the organism's characteristics and laboratory diagnosis
(ii) pathogenesis and clinical characteristics
(iii) epidemiology
(iv) prevention and, to a lesser degree, therapy

The cases were chosen for one of two reasons: they represented either typical presentations of infections due to commonly encountered organisms, or life-threatening or fatal infections with less frequently encountered organisms.

The material in this book has been written to supplement a traditional medical microbiology lecture course. This case-based learning approach may be used in small groups, in which the teacher's role is to lead the discussion of the important teaching points as outlined in the synopsis of each case. An extensive glossary is included here to explain much of the medical terminology, so that the cases should be accessible to nonclinical scientists, both teachers and students.

This book has three secondary goals. One is to help the students learn how to develop a differential diagnosis. The second is to help the student begin to understand the language of medicine. Access to a medical dictionary and a standard medical microbiology/infectious disease text will be very useful.

Third, this book is meant to be enjoyed. We hope the students will find solving these cases a satisfying and enriching learning experience.

This book was written as a supplement to the many excellent medical microbiology texts available, some of which are listed below.

Baron, S., *Medical Microbiology*, 3rd ed., Churchill-Livingstone, New York, 1991.
Davis, B. D., R. Dulbecco, H. N. Eisen, and H. S. Ginsberg, *Microbiology*, 4th ed., J. B. Lippincott, Philadelphia, 1990.
Jawetz, E., J. L. Melnick, and E. A. Adelberg, *Review of Medical Microbiology*, 19th ed., Appleton & Lange, East Norwalk, Conn., 1991.

Joklik, W. K., H. P. Willett, D. B. Amos, and C. M. Wilfert, *Zinsser Microbiology,* 20th ed., Appleton & Lange, East Norwalk, Conn., 1992.

Levinson, W. E., and E. Jawetz, *Medical Microbiology and Immunology: Examination and Board Review,* 2nd ed., Appleton & Lange, East Norwalk, Conn., 1992.

Schaechter, M., G. Medoff, and D. Schlessinger, *Mechanisms of Microbial Disease,* Williams & Wilkins, Baltimore, 1989.

Sherris, J. C., J. J. Champoux, L. Corey, F. C. Neidhardt, J. J. Plorde, C. G. Ray, and K. J. Ryan, *Medical Microbiology: An Introduction to Infectious Disease,* Elsevier, New York, 1990.

Volk, W. A., D. C. Benjamin, R. J. Kadner, and J. T. Parsons, *Essentials of Medical Microbiology,* 4th ed., J. B. Lippincott, Philadelphia, 1991.

Shulman, S. T., J. P. Phair, and H. M. Sommers, *The Biologic and Clinical Basis of Infectious Diseases,* 4th ed., W. B. Saunders, Philadelphia, 1992.

TO THE STUDENT

This text was written for you. It is an attempt to help you better understand the clinical importance of the basic science concepts you learn either in your medical microbiology lecture or through your independent study. You may also find that this text is useful in reviewing for Part I of the National Board of Medical Examiners exam. It should also be a good reference during your Infectious Disease rotations.

Below is a sample case, followed by a discussion of how you should approach a case to determine its likely etiology.

Sample case

A 6-year-old child presented with a 24-hour history of fever, vomiting, and complaining of a sore throat. On physical examination, she had a temperature of 38.5°C, her tonsillar region appeared inflamed and was covered by an exudate, and she had several enlarged cervical lymph nodes. A throat culture plated on sheep blood agar grew many beta-hemolytic colonies. These colonies were small with a comparatively wide zone of hemolysis.

What is the likely etiologic agent of her infection?

The first thing that should be done is to determine what type of infection this child has. She tells you that she has a sore throat. On physical exam, she has signs of an inflamed pharynx with exudate, which are consistent with her symptoms. (Do you know what an exudate is? If not, it's time to consult the glossary in the back of this text.) She also has enlarged regional lymph nodes, which support your diagnosis of pharyngitis (sore throat).

What is the etiology of her infection? The obvious response is that she has a "strep throat," but in reality there are many agents which can cause a clinical syndrome indistinguishable from that produced by group A streptococci, the etiologic agent of "strep throat." For example, sore throats are much more frequently caused by viruses than streptococci. Other bacteria can cause pharyngitis as well, including mycoplasma, various *Corynebacterium* spp., *Arcanobacterium*, and *Neisseria gonorrhoeae*. All of these organisms would be in the differential diagnosis, along with other perhaps more obscure causes of pharyngitis.

However, further laboratory information narrows the differential diagnosis considerably; small colonies that are surrounded by large zones of hemolysis are consistent with beta-hemolytic streptococci, specifically group A streptococci. Based on the presenting signs and symptoms and the laboratory data, this child most likely has group A streptococcal pharyngitis.

Specific aids have been added to the book to assist you in solving the cases.

1. At the end of each book section is a list of organisms. Only organisms on this list should be considered when solving the preceding cases. These lists have been organized on the basis of important characteristics of the listed organisms.
2. A table of normal values is available at the end of the text. If you are unsure whether a specific laboratory or vital sign finding is abnormal, consult this table.
3. A glossary of medical terms which are frequently used in the cases is available at the end of the text. If you do not understand a specific medical term, consult the glossary. If the term is not present there, you will have to consult a medical dictionary or other medical texts.
4. A key to the figures is provided at the end of the text. Consult it only if you are unable to solve those cases which refer to a specific figure.

Some final thoughts

1. Microscopic descriptions of the organism are given in many of the cases so you can narrow your differential diagnosis. Use them.

2. The temptation for many will be to read the case and its accompanying questions and then go directly to reading the answers. You will derive more benefit from this text by working through the questions and subsequently reading the case discussion.

Have fun and good luck!

ACKNOWLEDGMENTS

This project became a reality through the assistance of many individuals. We first would like to recognize the students of the 1994 and 1995 classes of the University of North Carolina School of Medicine. Their enthusiasm for this case-based teaching approach provided momentum for our undertaking of this project. We thank our fellow faculty involved in the medical microbiology course at UNC for their willingness to have us pilot this new innovative teaching approach. We thank Drs. Harry Gooder, Roy Hopfer, and Jean Bowdre for their critiques of selected cases. We appreciate the careful reviews by Drs. Philip Coyne and Rick Hodinka as well as by the ASM Books' reviewers, including Dr. Martha Mulks, Michigan State University; Dr. N. Cary Engleberg, University of Michigan Medical School; Dr. Patrick Schlievert, University of Minnesota Medical School; Dr. David Welch, University of Oklahoma Medical School; Dr. Richard Hyde, University of Oklahoma Medical School; Dr. Roberta Carey, St. Francis Hospital; Dr. Karin Mcgowan, University of Pennsylvania Medical School; and Dr. Ted Schutzbank, Children's National Medical Center and George Washington University. We thank Dr. Jim Folds for his support during the preparation of this book and his review of selected cases. Any errors or shortcomings in the book are entirely our own.

We appreciate the assistance of Drs. Janet Fischer and Margaret Johnson in contributing some case material. Dr. Fischer's encyclopedic knowledge of cases seen at our medical center was invaluable.

We want to thank Will Owens for the excellent photography and Dr. T. Paul Walden for preparation of the glossary. We are indebted to our secretaries, Karen Alston, Sharon Linville, and Leigh Noble, for their patience, good humor, and diligence throughout the preparation of this book. We thank Mary Farrell for successfully locating several hundred medical records during our selection of the final cases used in the text. We also would like to thank Jill, Claudia, and Robert Shapiro for their patience and support during this project.

Finally, we would like to acknowledge Ellie Tupper, senior production editor, and Yvonne Strong, copy editor, for their excellent contributions, and Pat Fitzgerald for his unflagging enthusiasm and support for the publication of this book.

BACTERIOLOGY

This text begins with cases involving bacterial pathogens. Bacterial infections tend to be more familiar to the beginning student. Many of you will have had personal experience with bacterial infections such as "strep throat," urinary tract infections, or superficial wound infections. This is the only section of the text where a conscious effort has been made to go from easier to more difficult cases. It is also true that certain questions are asked repeatedly. This is done to emphasize specific facts and concepts which we feel are important for you to know. An attempt has been made to organize the cases by types of infection so that cases of meningitis, diarrheal disease, and sexually transmitted disease are each grouped together. Specific antimicrobial therapy is discussed only in those cases where a clear consensus exists. The student should understand that standard antimicrobial therapy constantly evolves, especially for organisms which are very adaptable at developing antimicrobial resistance such as *Pseudomonas aeruginosa*.

A mixture of community- and noscomially acquired infections has been included. Frequently encountered pathogens are emphasized, but cases due to infrequently encountered pathogens which demonstrate important medical microbiology concepts are also presented. Finally, the changing epidemiology and disease spectrum of bacterial pathogens in the era of AIDS and widespread organ transplantation is addressed.

The patient was a 15-year-old male with a history of sickle cell disease. He presented on the morning of hospital admission with a 4-day history of a progressive, productive cough and 2 days of spiking fevers. On admission, his temperature was 41.1°C, his respiratory rate was 40/min, pulse was 120 beats/min, and his blood pressure was 80/40 mmHg. He was alert and in mild respiratory distress. Chest examination was notable for decreased breath sounds by auscultation and dullness to percussion. Initial laboratory studies included a hematocrit of 13.6% and a white blood cell (leukocyte; WBC) count of 52,400/mm^3 with 86% neutrophils. A sputum Gram stain was non-diagnostic. A chest radiograph demonstrated a right lower lobe infiltrate. A blood culture was subsequently positive for gram-positive cocci in pairs (diplococci). (See Figure 1.)

1. What is the clinical diagnosis in this patient? Was the sputum Gram stain an appropriate test in this case?

2. What is the likely organism causing this illness? What is the major virulence factor of this organism?

3. Patients with sickle cell disease are at increased risk for bacterial infections with what types of organisms? Why?

4. Name two possible ways of preventing bacterial pneumonia in sickle cell patients.

DISCUSSION

1. This patient had community-acquired bacterial pneumonia on the basis of his physical examination and chest radiograph. The presence of decreased breath sounds, dullness to percussion, and lung opacity on radiograph are consistent with the presence of fluid in his alveoli. The extraordinarily high white blood cell count of 52,400 with significantly elevated numbers of neutrophils strongly supported the diagnosis of an infection, specifically a bacterial pneumonia. In this patient, the Gram stain was not diagnostic. However, in many patients with bacterial pneumonia and bronchitis, the sputum Gram stain can be extremely valuable in guiding empirical therapy.

2. The most common cause of community-acquired bacterial pneumonia is *Streptococcus pneumoniae.* The finding of gram-positive diplococci in the blood is consistent with pneumococcal disease as well. Approximately 25 to 30% of patients with pneumococcal pneumonia will have positive blood cultures. Group A streptococcus is another possible organism because it can cause bacteremic pneumonia and can possibly appear as a gram-positive diplococcus. However, in a blood culture, group A streptococci are much more likely to be present as gram-positive cocci in chains. The two streptococci are easily distinguished by the fact that *S. pneumoniae* is alpha-hemolytic and bile soluble whereas group A streptococcus is beta-hemolytic and bile insoluble but bacitracin susceptible.

    The major virulence factor of *S. pneumoniae* is a polysaccharide capsule. This capsule is antiphagocytic, promoting the survival of this organism in the lungs. There are more than 80 antigenically distinct capsular types (serotypes), although certain serotypes (serotypes 3, 6, 19, and 23) are more commonly isolated. Strains posessing certain polysaccharides (type 3, for example) are believed to be more virulent than other strains with different capsular types.

3. Patients with sickle cell anemia are at a greatly increased risk of infection with encapsulated organisms including pneumococci, *Haemophilus influenzae* type b, *Neisseria meningitidis,* and *Salmonella enteriditis.* Besides pneumonia, bacteremia, and meningitis, osteomyelitis primarily due to *Salmonella* spp. is a problem in these patients. Patients with sickle cell anemia are functionally asplenic because early in life they have splenic infarcts due to the sludging of sickle cells in the splenic circulation. They can have a defective alternative complement pathway and be deficient in serum opsonic activity. All of these factors contribute to their increased susceptibility to encapsulated bacterial organisms. In particular, a major

splenic function is to filter encapsulated organisms from the blood, and this capability is defective in this patient population.

4. Immunization with the current pneumococcal vaccine (which contains polysaccharide antigens from 23 *S. pneumoniae* serotypes) may provide protective antibodies to many of the common pneumococcal isolates.

Prophylactic oral penicillin, which is not entirely without risks, provides some protection against bacteria which are sensitive to this antibiotic. The pneumococci are generally susceptible to penicillin so that this regimen should provide adequate protection against pneumococcal pneumonia.

REFERENCES

Jorgensen, J. H., A. W. Howell, L. A. Maher, and R. R. Facklam. 1991. Serotypes of respiratory isolates of *Streptococcus pneumoniae* compared with capsular types included in the current pneumococcal vaccine. *J. Infect. Dis.* **163:**644–646.

Pearson, H. A., R. P. Spencer, and E. A. Cornelius. 1969. Functional asplenia in sickle cell anemia. *N. Engl. J. Med.* **281:**923–927.

The patient was a 43-year-old female with a history of mitral valve prolapse. She was admitted with a chief complaint of intermittent fevers for 1 month and headaches for 3 weeks. Two weeks prior to developing symptoms, she had undergone a dental procedure for which she took prophylactic erythromycin (she was penicillin allergic). She had no skin lesions or hemorrhages in the nail beds. All four blood cultures performed on admission were positive for gram-positive cocci in chains.

1. What is your diagnosis?

2. Which organism is most likely to be causing her infection? What is the likely source of the organism?

3. Why did she receive prophylactic antimicrobial agents before dental procedures?

4. Which organs often become secondarily infected in this infection? What are septic emboli, and what role do they have in these secondary infections?

DISCUSSION

1. The diagnosis in this patient is difficult. The patient's chief complaints were somewhat vague, but the observation that they occurred soon after a dental procedure in someone with a heart valve abnormality suggests that the patient might have had bacterial endocarditis. The diagnosis of bacterial endocarditis was further supported by the finding that all four blood cultures were positive.

2. The description of gram-positive cocci in chains suggests that the organisms are streptococci. Two groups of streptococci are common causes of bacterial endocarditis. They are viridans streptococci (the so-called alpha-hemolytic or "green" streptococci) and nonhemolytic streptococci (which include group D streptococci and the enterococci). Because the individual had recently undergone a dental procedure, the organism causing the infection probably represents the oral flora rather than the gut flora. The group D streptococci and enterococci are commonly found as part of the normal flora in the gut, whereas viridans streptocci are common members of the oral flora. *Streptococcus mutans,* a viridans streptococcus, was the organism recovered from this patient. It commonly resides on the tongue and teeth.

3. In people with heart valve anomalies, prophylactic antimicrobial agents are commonly used prior to dental procedures. The rationale for their use is that during dental procedures, transient bacteremia occurs in up to 80% of individuals. (Transient bacteremia is defined as the presence of bacteria in the bloodstream for short periods. The organisms which cause this are generally of low virulence and are usually easily removed from the bloodstream by the reticuloendothelial system.) The organisms which commonly cause this bacteremia are oral streptococci, which readily adhere to a variety of surfaces. In particular, abnormal heart valves may become infected by these "sticky" organisms. Vegetations may form and then endocarditis develops.

4. Septic emboli (i.e., blood clots containing bacteria) are often produced in bacterial endocarditis. These emboli are shed into the bloodstream from the infected heart valve. They enter the circulation and can become lodged in blood vessels throughout the body. Abscess formation due to these septic emboli occurs most frequently in the brain, but also is seen in the organs of the reticuloendothelial system (spleen, liver) and the kidneys. Petechial skin lesions are seen in 20 to 40% of patients with endocarditis and can be the result of septic emboli.

REFERENCES

Roberts, R. B., A. G. Krieger, and N. L. Schiller. 1979. Viridans streptococcal endocarditis: the role of various species including pyridoxal-dependent streptococci. *Rev. Infect. Dis.* 1:955–966.
Scheld, W. M., O. Zak, K. Vosbeck, and M. A. Sande. 1981. Bacterial adhesion in the
pathogenesis of infective endocarditis. *J. Clin. Invest.* 68:1381–1384.

The patient was a 23-year-old female with an autoimmune connective tissue disorder who presented with fever, left foot and right upper quadrant pain, nausea, and vomiting. An exploratory laparatomy was performed during which 300 ml of greenish, nonodorous purulent material was aspirated from the peritoneum. An appendectomy was performed as well. The aspirate of the peritoneum revealed moderate polymorphonuclear leukocytes (PMNs) and few gram-positive cocci. Aspirate of the fourth metatarsal joint revealed numerous PMNs, but no organisms were seen. An admission blood culture and joint and peritoneal aspirates grew the same organism, which was very mucoid and beta-hemolytic.

1. When colonies are mucoid, this usually indicates the presence of which virulence factor?

2. Which three types of infections does this patient have?

3. On the basis of Gram stain and the infections observed, this organism belongs to which genus?

4. What further characteristics of this organism would be helpful in determining its identity?

The technologist returned the organism to the incubator after doing the tests suggested by you in your response to question 4, noting that the colonies were very mucoid. She took the culture out of the incubator 5 h later to show the infectious disease fellow, telling her that "you should see how mucoid this organism is!" When she showed the fellow the plate, the colonies were no longer mucoid. (See Figure 2.)

5. Explain the observation just described.

6. What organism is this? Comment on the epidemiology of systemic infections with this organism.

DISCUSSION

1. Mucoid colonies are generally encapsulated.

2. The patient had septic arthritis (white cells and organisms in a joint), peritonitis (organisms and pus in the peritoneum), and bacteremia (bacteria in the bloodstream). All of these body sites are usually sterile.

3. The two most common gram-positive cocci which could be responsible for the infections described above are the staphylococci and the streptococci. Because the organism is beta-hemolytic, it is likely to be either a *Staphylococcus aureus* isolate or a beta-hemolytic streptococcus.

4. Streptococci can be easily distinguished from staphylococci on the basis of a catalase test: streptococci are catalase negative, and *S. aureus* are catalase positive. The arrangement of the organism on Gram stain would also be very helpful in determining whether the infectious agent in this case is a streptococcus (gram-positive cocci in chains) or a staphylococcus (gram-positive cocci in clusters). If the organism is catalase positive, a coagulase test would be used to determine whether it is *S. aureus* (coagulase positive). If it is catalase negative, serogrouping could be used to determine the group to which the organism belongs.

5 and 6. The organism causing this infection is a group A streptococcus. The mucoid phenotype of this organism is due to the production of a hyaluronic acid capsule. Group A streptococci also produce the enzyme hyaluronidase, which can degrade this capsule. During the 5-h incubation, the organism began to hydrolyze its capsule. As a result of the degraded capsule, the colonies were no longer mucoid.

   In the past 3 to 5 years there has been a resurgence in serious group A streptococcal infections. We see several cases of group A streptococcal bacteremia and serious wound infections each year at our institution. There has been a temporal relationship between this resurgence and the appearance of mucoid strains of group A streptococci. A series of systemic group A streptococcal infections associated with a toxic shock-like syndrome have recently been reported. The mortality rate in this study was 30%. Only one of the isolates studied was mucoid, but 8 of 10 produced pyrogenic exotoxin A, also called the scarlet fever toxin.

REFERENCE

Stevens, D. L., M. H. Tanner, J. Winship, R. Swartz, K. M. Ries, P. M. Schlievert, and E. Kaplan. 1989. Severe group A streptococcal infections associated with a toxic shock-like syndrome and scarlet fever toxin A. *N. Engl. J. Med.* **321**:1–6.

This 53-year-old woman had a medical history notable for significant pelvic trauma 14 months prior to hospital admission. Since that time, she has failed conservative management of severe urinary incontinence. Her medical history was otherwise significant for multiple recurrent urinary tract infections (including *Escherichia coli*, *Pseudomonas aeruginosa*, and *Proteus mirabilis* infections) that had been treated with courses of antibiotics. The patient was admitted and underwent urologic and gynecologic surgery. She received prophylactic doses of cefoxitin, a cephalosporin, during the 24-h perioperative period. Two days postoperatively, the patient developed a fever to 39°C and some abdominal tenderness. Blood cultures drawn at the time of the fever were subsequently positive for gram-positive cocci.

1. Which organisms are likely to be responsible for her bacteremia?

2. Subsequent biochemical tests demonstrated that the isolate was catalase negative, bile-esculin positive, and able to grow in 6.5% NaCl. Which organism is this?

3. Is this organism part of the normal bacterial flora? If so, where?

4. Which types of infections does this organism cause?

5. In which types of patients do infections with this organism tend to occur?

6. In serious infections with this organism (in particular, endocarditis), ampicillin is often given in combination with an aminoglycoside such as gentamicin or streptomycin. What is the rational basis (in vitro) for this decision?

DISCUSSION

1. Because of the temporal relationship between the surgery and the development of abdominal tenderness and fevers, it is likely that her infection was secondary to her surgery. Organisms likely to cause bacteremia following genitourinary (GU) tract surgery would include members of the normal flora in the genitourinary tract. These are very diverse and include staphylococci; various species of streptococci and enterococci; many different types of anaerobes including *Bacteroides, Peptostreptococcus, Fusobacterium, Bifidobacterium, Clostridium,* and *Mobiluncus* species; yeasts; lactobacilli, diphtheroids, *Gardnerella* spp.; and, in some individuals, members of the family *Enterobacteriaceae.* Because the patient received a prophylactic antimicrobial agent, many of these organisms, owing to their susceptibility, become less likely. Because gram-positive cocci were recovered from the blood, the list of possible organisms causing this infection can be narrowed considerably to include streptococci, enterococci, staphylococci, and peptostreptococci.

2. On the basis of the biochemical tests cited here, this organism belongs to the genus *Enterococcus.* Species which commonly cause human infection are *Enterococcus faecalis* (most frequent) and *E. faecium.*

3. The enterococci are members of the normal flora of the human gastrointestinal tract, reaching concentrations of 10^7 to 10^9 CFU/g in the feces of normal adults. They also can be present in the genitourinary tract, skin, and oropharynx, although they may be isolated less frequently and at fairly low concentrations at the last two sites.

4 and 5. Enterococci can cause a variety of types of infections in a number of different types of patients. They are the most common etiologic agents of urinary tract infection caused by gram-positive organisms. They are particulary important as a cause of nosocomial urinary tract infections in patients with indwelling catheters. They are a common cause of endocarditis in patients with abnormal or prosthetic heart valves. They can infect a wide array of indwelling lines and devices, probably because of an ability to adhere to these foreign bodies. They are frequently isolated along with multiple other organisms in intra-abdominal abscesses. Their pathogenic role in abscess formation is probably secondary. They are frequently associated with wound infections, especially in patients receiving broad-spectrum antimicrobial agents, to which enterococci are frequently resistant. In fact, in patients receiving broad-spectrum antimicrobial agents, enterococci are major causes of nosocomial infections of the urinary tract, bloodstream, and wounds.

6. In serious infections, the antimicrobial therapy used should be rapidly bactericidal if at all possible. Ampicillin when used alone inhibits the growth of enterococci in vitro but kills them extremely slowly or not at all. The aminoglycosides streptomycin and gentamicin will not inhibit the in vitro growth of enterococci. This is because the aminoglycosides cannot penetrate into the cytoplasm of enterococci to their target, the ribosomes. However, when concentrations of ampicillin and aminoglycosides achievable in the bloodstream are mixed in a test tube with enterococci, the organisms are killed rapidly. When a combination of two antimicrobial agents kills an organism much more rapidly than does either agent alone, this phenomenon is known as synergy. In patients with enterococcal endocarditis, using antimicrobial combinations which are synergistic in vitro has a better clinical outcome than using ampicillin alone. The synergy is believed to occur because ampicillin causes alterations in the cell membrane of the enterococci, allowing transport of the aminoglycosides into the cell.

REFERENCES

Herman, D. J., and D. N. Gerding. 1991. Screening and treatment of infections caused by resistant enterococci. *Antimicrob. Agents Chemother.* **35:**215–218.

Matusumoto, J. Y., W. R. Wilson, A. J. Wright, J. E. Geraci, and J. A. Washington II. 1980. Synergy of penicillin and decreasing concentrations of aminoglycosides against enterococci from patients with infective endocarditis. *Antimicrob. Agents Chemother.* **18:**944–947.

This 8-year-old boy developed spiking fevers 1 week prior to hospital admission. The fever was treated with acetaminophen and ibuprofen. He also complained of right ankle pain and anterior tibial tenderness that was attributed to summer sports activities although he did not have any known injury to the extremity. Two days prior to admission he presented for evaluation. At that time he had mild distal tibial tenderness, no ankle effusion, a normal white blood cell count, an erythrocyte sedimentation rate of 55 mm/h (normal 0 to 15 mm/h), and normal radiographs of the ankle and tibia. The patient was thought to have a viral syndrome and was sent home. On the day of his admission to the hospital, he developed severe pain and tenderness in the right leg and a fever of 39.4°C. Radiographs were again negative.

An ankle aspiration revealed fluid with 3,350 WBC/mm^3 with 86% neutrophils. A bone scan was reportedly "hot" in the right distal tibia. Bacterial cultures of blood, fluid from the ankle joint, and tibial aspirate were all positive for the same organism, which on Gram stain appears as gram-positive cocci. (See Figure 3.)

1. Which organisms would be consistent with the Gram stain and the case presentation?

2. The organism was subsequently found to be both catalase and coagulase positive. What is this organism?

3. Where in nature is this bacterium found? How do people become infected?

4. This patient has osteomyelitis and septic arthritis. Name two ways in which bacteria may invade bone and joints to cause these infections. How is this type of infection managed?

5. What other types of infections does this organism cause?

DISCUSSION

1 and 2. Two major genera of bacteria would be likely in this particular case, staphylococci and streptococci. The arrangement of the organism on Gram stain would be helpful in determining the genus to which this organism belonged. In clinical specimens, staphylococci tend to appear in clusters while streptococci appear either as diploids or in chains. These arrangements occur because streptococci divide only in a single plane whereas staphylococci can divide in multiple ones. Direct Gram stain results can be useful in guiding initial antimicrobial therapy before the infecting agent has been isolated and identified. Once isolated, staphylococci can be easily distinguished from streptococci on the basis of colony morphology, hemolytic reactions, and the catalase test, staphylococci being catalase positive and streptococci being catalase negative. If the organism is a catalase-positive, gram-positive coccus, a coagulase test is performed. Coagulase-positive organisms have the ability to clot rabbit plasma. Organisms unable to do this are considered coagulase negative. Only one *Staphylococcus* species which infects humans is coagulase positive: *Staphylococcus aureus. S. aureus* is the most frequent cause of osteomyelitis. There are more than 20 different species of coagulase-negative staphylococci, with *S. epidermidis* and *S. saprophyticus* being the 2 most important. *S. epidermidis* causes a variety of infections, almost all of which are related to foreign bodies. *S. saprophyticus* causes urinary tract infections primarily in young, sexually active women.

3. *S. aureus* is carried in the nares of approximately 20 to 40% of adults. From the nares, the organism can be transferred to the skin. Carriers of the organism can pass it to others, usually by direct contact or by droplets. This is believed to be the primary way in which nosocomial (hospital-acquired) wound infections occur. Infections can also occur when the organism penetrates the skin following trauma. This trauma can be inapparent.

4. There are two mechanisms by which patients can develop osteomyelitis and septic arthritis. One is hematogenous spread of the organism. In this scenario, the organism invades the site of infection during bacteremia. In such cases, there often is local trauma at the site of infection with compromise of the vasculature, providing an ideal environment for infection. The second way is by invasion of the bone and joint from a contiguous site of infection. This individual may have had a superficial wound infection with *S. aureus* secondary to trauma from his athletic activities. The organism then invaded the joint and/or bone directly from this wound. In both hematogenous and contiguous spread of the organism to bone and joint, trauma plays an important role. Osteomyelitis can also be a complication

of surgery, especially orthopedic procedures. It is particularly problematic after knee and hip replacement surgery.

Most patients are managed conservatively with long-term antimicrobial therapy. In addition, areas of pus such as the septic joint or abscesses should be drained because antimicrobial agents penetrate poorly into these sites of infection. Certain antimicrobial agents have reduced activity in pus because of its low pH or its anaerobic conditions.

5. *S. aureus* causes a wide array of infections. Its versatility is largely due to its ability to accommodate the genetic information of a wide array of virulence factors. It can cause localized skin infections such as folliculitis, carbuncles, furuncles, and impetigo. It can also cause localized infections with systemic manifestations due to the production of exotoxins. Two examples are staphylococcal scalded skin syndrome, during which the organism produces an exfoliative toxin that causes separation of large areas of the epidermis from the dermis. This desquamation leads to the scalded appearance of the skin from which this syndrome gets its name. This disease is seen primarily in infants. Another localized infection with systemic complications is toxic shock syndrome. Again, the manifestations of this disease are primarily due to the activity of an exotoxin called toxic shock syndrome toxin-1. It should be emphasized that only certain strains of *S. aureus* produce either one of these two toxins; many produce neither.

S. *aureus* can also cause bacteremia and its severe complication, endocarditis. It can also produce abscesses at many sites throughout the body. Of special concern is its ability to cause pulmonary superinfection in patients with influenza virus pneumonia. The interaction of these two agents is manifested by multiple lung abscesses. Finally, certain strains of *S. aureus* which produce enterotoxins can cause food poisoning. Food poisoning is often a result of contamination of high-protein foods such as dairy and meat products by food preparers who carry these enterotoxin-producing *S. aureus* strains on their hands or in their nares.

REFERENCES

Cohen, M. L. 1986. *Staphylococcus aureus*: biology, mechanism of virulence, epidemiology. *J. Pediatr.* 5:796–799.

Nelson, J. D. 1990. Acute ostemomyelitis in children. *Infect. Dis. Clin. N. Am.* 4:513–522.

This 47-year-old man had a history of sickle cell disease that resulted in many previous hospitalizations for the management of painful crisis. Owing to multiple hospitalizations requiring the placement of intravenous lines, the patient had poor peripheral venous access, and a right port-a-cath (a central venous catheter that is designed to remain in place for a prolonged period) was placed in his right subclavian vein.

The patient was admitted 9 days prior to the current admission for the management of a painful crisis. His pain was successfully managed, and he was discharged after a 4-day hospitalization. On the day of readmission, the patient noted the presence of right arm discomfort and swelling, a temperature of 38.1°C, and chills. He presented to the hospital emergency room, where he was afebrile. Physical examination was remarkable for right upper extremity swelling.

A Doppler sonographic examination of the venous system of his right upper extremity demonstrated right axillary and right subclavian venous thromboses. Blood cultures were obtained (one set through the port-a-cath and one set via a peripheral vein). The two sets of blood cultures grew identical gram-positive cocci.

1. Which organisms are most likely to cause this infection? Of these, which is the most common?

2. What is the major virulence factor of the organism causing this infection?

3. What risk factor does this patient have which predisposes him to infection with this organism?

4. What is the significance of his two positive blood cultures?

5. Which other types of culture besides blood would be useful in determining his specific type of infection?

DISCUSSION

1. On the basis of this patient's blood culture results and the presence of a foreign body, the staphylococci and streptococci are the most likely agents of his infection. This patient in all likelihood (see the discussion of questions 4 and 5 for further explanation) had line-related sepsis. The most common causes of line-related infection are the staphylococci, with the coagulase-negative staphylococci being more frequently recovered than *Staphylococcus aureus*. With the introduction and widespread use of intravascular prosthetic devices made of synthetic materials, the coagulase-negative staphylococci have become the most important cause of nosocomial bactemia, with these devices acting as the source of the bacteremia. There are in excess of 20 species of coagulase-negative staphylococci. Most laboratories do not identify these organisms to the species level, preferring to report them simply as coagulase-negative staphylococci. The exception to this is in urinary tract infections, when *S. saprophyticus* can be presumptively identified from its susceptibility to novobiocin. It is an important cause of urinary tract infection in young, sexually active women. Other common species of coagulase-negative staphylococci include the most commonly recovered species, *S. epidermidis*, as well as *S. hominis, S. haemolyticus, S. warneri, S. simulans,* and *S. cohnii.*

   Another organism which must also be considered in this case is *Streptococcus pneumoniae* because of its high frequency of infection in patients with sickle cell disease. This organism is rarely seen as a cause of line-related sepsis, however. The organism recovered from this patient was a coagulase-negative staphylococcus.

2. Species of coagulase-negative staphylococci produce a virulence factor referred to as slime. Slime has been shown to enhance the adherence of stapylococci to a wide variety of plastic surfaces. Slime-producing strains of coagulase-negative staphylococci may be more difficult to eradicate by antimicrobial therapy than non-slime-producing ones.

3. Coagulase-negative staphylococci are normal inhabitants of the skin, mucous membranes, and nares. Any indwelling device introduced through the skin places an individual at risk for infection with this organism. The presence of a port-a-cath in this patient is an important risk factor for his development of this infection.

4 and 5. The diagnosis of line-related sepsis is made by first obtaining two blood cultures from a patient who develops fever and, in some instances, by observing localized signs of infection at the site of the intravascular line. One of the blood cultures is obtained through the line, and the other

is obtained from a peripheral site. The reason for requiring cultures drawn from two sites is fairly straightforward. Since coagulase-negative staphylococci are commonly found on the skin and are the most frequent cause of blood culture contamination, a single positive blood culture with this organism may represent skin contamination rather than true infection. However, if blood cultures obtained from two separate sites grow the same organism, it is more likely that the recovery of this organism represents infection rather than contamination. In addition, if the peripheral blood culture is negative for coagulase-negative staphylococci and the culture drawn through the line is positive, this may represent local infection of the catheter site. In such a situation the catheter site should be fully examined for signs of infection, such as erythema and tenderness.

The diagnosis of line-related sepsis can be confirmed by performing a semiquantitative culture on the catheter tip. The culture is done by aseptically removing the catheter, cutting off the tip with sterile scissors, and transporting it to the laboratory for culture. In the laboratory, the tip is rolled on the surface of an agar plate. After appropriate incubation, the number of colonies present on the plate is counted. If 15 CFU of a single or multiple species is present per plate and the blood cultures are positive, the patient is said to have catheter- or line-related sepsis. This infection is best treated by catheter removal and antimicrobial therapy.

REFERENCES

Maki, D. G., C. E. Weise, and H. W. Sarafin. 1977. A semi-quantitative method for identifying intravenous-catheter-related infection. *N. Engl. J. Med.* **296:**1305–1309.

Younger, J. J., G. D. Christsen, D. L. Bartley, J. C. H. Simmons, and F. F. Barett. 1987. Coagulase-negative staphylococci isolated from cerebrospinal fluid shunts: importance of slime production, species identification and shunt removal to clinical outcome. *J. Infect. Dis.* **156:**548–554.

This 6-year-old female presented with a 1-week history of a febrile illness with a sore throat and headache. She was given oral ampicillin by her local physician. One day prior to hospital admission, the patient awakened with pain and swelling in the right ankle. She was evaluated on the day of admission, and in addition to a warm, swollen right ankle, she was noted to have a new grade III/VI systolic heart murmur thought to be consistent with mitral regurgitation (insufficiency of the mitral valve). She was admitted to the hospital with a presumptive diagnosis of acute rheumatic fever.

1. The patient had a sore throat that preceded her acute rheumatic fever. Although we do not have the results of a throat culture taken during the sore throat, which pathogen would probably have grown from such a culture? How can an "A" disc (which contains bacitracin) help in the identification of this organism?

2. How is pharyngitis with this bacterium related to the subsequent development of rheumatic fever?

3. Which type of hemolysis is seen when this organism is streaked on sheep blood agar? Which types of hemolysins does this bacteria make?

4. Which serologic test may be useful in helping to confirm the diagnosis of rheumatic fever in this patient?

5. Which cell wall protein is believed to play a major role in the pathogenesis of rheumatic fever? Explain its role specifically.

6. Is the incidence of rheumatic fever increasing in the United States? Explain your answer.

7. What is scarlet fever? Is it related to rheumatic fever?

DISCUSSION

1 and 2. Rheumatic fever is a nonsuppurative sequela of *Streptococcus pyogenes* (group A streptococcus) infection. It occurs approximately 3 weeks (range, 1 to 5 weeks) after group A streptococcal pharyngitis. At the time of development of the symptoms of rheumatic fever, throat cultures for group A streptococci are often negative. A recent history of group A streptococcal pharyngitis, however, supports the diagnosis of rheumatic fever. In this case, the patient had a history of a sore throat and presumably had group A streptococcal pharyngitis. It should be noted that viral pharyngitis occurs at least as frequently as group A streptococcal pharyngitis. The finding of a sore throat without culture confirmation of *S. pyogenes* infection, then, is of limited value in establishing the diagnosis of rheumatic fever.

   The "A" disc is a diagnostic test for the presumptive identification of group A streptococci. The growth of *S. pyogenes* usually is inhibited by bacitracin, whereas the growth of other beta-hemolytic streptococci usually is not. The identification is only presumptive because the growth of 3 to 5% of the *S. pyogenes* strains is not inhibited by this compound, whereas the growth of a small number (5 to 10%) of beta-hemolytic group B, C, and G streptococci is inhibited by it.

3. *S. pyogenes* is a beta-hemolytic organism. (See Figure 2.) It produces two distinct hemolysins, streptolysin S and streptolysin O. Both can lyse a variety of cell types, including red blood cells. Streptolysin O is a potent hemolysin, but it is oxygen labile. (Streptolysin S is oxygen stable.) To demonstrate the presence of streptolysin O, throat specimens streaked on blood agar plates are frequently stabbed with the inoculating loop so that colonies of group A streptococci can grow beneath the agar surface and produce this hemolysin under "anaerobic" conditions.

4. Patients with rheumatic fever frequently (80%) mount a humoral immune response to streptolysin O. The test used to measure antibody levels against this hemolysin is called an ASO (anti-streptolysin O) titer. An elevated ASO titer in individuals with appropriate clinical symptoms supports the diagnosis of rheumatic fever. The diagnosis of rheumatic fever is a clinical one with established diagnostic criteria (the revised Jones criteria).

5. M protein is an important virulence factor found in the cell wall of virulent strains of *S. pyogenes*. This virulence factor has been found to be antiphagocytic. It also has epitopes which are antigenically similar to ones found in cardiac myosin and sarcolemmal membrane proteins. The conventional wisdom concerning acute rheumatic fever is that it is an auto-

immune disease. It is believed that antibodies directed against the M protein cross-react with cardiac tissue. These antibodies bind to cross-reacting antigens in muscle and damage it. Other group A streptococcal antigens may also cross-react with other cardiac antigens, damaging other regions of the heart, such as the heart valves.

6. After many years of declining in the United States, the incidence of rheumatic fever has recently increased. Outbreaks have been seen among children in Utah and Ohio and military recruits in California. The reasons for the change in the epidemiology of this disease are unknown.

7. Scarlet fever is a manifestation of group A streptococcal pharyngitis in which the infecting strain produces a specific virulence factor called erythrogenic toxin, which is coded for by a phage. Production of this toxin is manifested clinically by the appearance of a scarlatinal (bright-red) rash beginning on the chest and spreading to the trunk and neck, and then to the extremities. The rash does not affect the face, palms, or soles. A "strawberry" tongue is frequently seen with this disease as well. Rheumatic fever can be a poststreptococcal sequela to scarlet fever, as it can be to streptococcal pharyngitis caused by strains which do not produce erythrogenic toxin.

Recently strains of group A streptococci which produce erythrogenic toxin have been associated with a toxic shock-like syndrome. This syndrome is associated with a high mortality (approximately 30%).

REFERENCES

American Heart Association. 1965. Jones Criteria (revised) for guidance in the diagnosis of acute rheumatic fever. *Circulation* **32:**664–668.

Veasy, L. G., S. E. Wiedmeier, G. S. Orsmond, H. D. Ruttenberg, M. M. Boucek, S. J. Roth, V. F. Tait, J. A. Thompson, J. A. Daly, E. L. Kaplan, and H. R. Hill. 1987. Resurgence of acute rheumatic fever in the Intermountain area of the United States. *N. Engl. J. Med.* **316:**421–427.

The patient was a 5½-week-old male who was transferred to our institution with a 10-day history of choking spells. The child's spells began with repetitive coughing, progressing to his turning red and gasping for breath. In the prior 2 days, he also had three episodes of vomiting in association with his choking spells. His physical examination was significant for a pulse of 160 beats/min and respiratory rate of 72 (both highly elevated). The child's chest radiograph was clear. There was no evidence of tracheal abnormalities. His white cell count was 15,500/mm³ with 70% lymphocytes. A nasopharyngeal swab was diagnostic.

1. What was the organism infecting this child?

2. Why is a nasopharyngeal swab the specimen of choice for making this diagnosis?

3. Why did this patient have a predominance of lymphocytes?

4. Are this child's clinical course and chest radiograph consistent with his infection? Explain your answer.

5. What is the epidemiology of this infection, and how might it be prevented?

DISCUSSION

1. This child had a classic presentation for whooping cough, whose etiologic agent is *Bordetella pertussis*.

2. The organism specifically binds to ciliated epithelial cells. This binding is mediated by filamentous hemagglutinin (FHA), an important virulence factor of this organism. Since the nasopharynx is lined with ciliated epithelial cells, culture of this site has a higher yield than any other specimen types.

3. *B. pertussis* produces a variety of virulence factors including pertussis toxin. In earlier literature, pertussis toxin was described as many different entities usually on the basis of a particular biological activity. One of the terms used to describe it was "lymphocytosis-promoting factor" because when injected into mice it was observed that 50% of the peripheral white blood cells were lymphocytes (normal approximately 25%). Clinically, lymphocytosis, often as high as 70 to 80%, is routinely seen in patients with whooping cough and is characteristic of this infection.

4. Yes. This child's presentation is typical of whooping cough. This infection is usually limited to the upper airways, and pneumonia due to either *B. pertussis* or secondary bacterial agents is unusual. Therefore, normal chest radiographs are common.

   Children with whooping cough often have paroxysms of coughing. The term "paroxysm" means a sudden recurrence or intensification. Children often cough repeatedly, and when they gasp for breath, the sound of this inspiration is the whoop of whooping cough. Because of repetitive coughing and resulting disruption of breathing, the children will have abnormal oxygen exchange and will often turn red and sometimes blue. The repetitive coughing may also result in vomiting or choking on respiratory secretions. All of these signs were seen in this child.

5. This disease is spread from person to person via respiratory secretions. No animal vector or reservoir has been identified. Young children, especially those under 2 months of age, are at increased risk for developing *B. pertussis*. At the age of 2 months a series of pertussis vaccinations is begun. Immunity increases with increasing numbers of doses of the vaccine, but the efficacy of the vaccine even after the entire series is probably no better than 90%. The disease is most severe in children under 6 months. When *B. pertussis* vaccination rates decline in the population, as has occurred in the past owing to reports of adverse effects of the vaccine, this population is the one most at peril.

REFERENCES

Pittman, M. 1979. Pertussis toxin: the cause of the harmful effects and prolonged immunity of whooping cough. A hypothesis. *Rev. Infect. Dis.* **1:**401–412.

Sato, Y., M. Kireura, and H. Fukuru. 1984. Development of a pertussis component vaccine in Japan. *Lancet* **i:**122–126.

This 2-year-old male child experienced an upper respiratory infection 2 weeks prior to hospital admission. Four days prior to admission, anorexia and lethargy were noted. The patient was seen in the emergency room 3 days prior to admission. At that time he had a fever of 39.9°C. Physical examination revealed a clear chest, exudative pharyngitis, and bilaterally enlarged cervical lymph nodes. A throat culture was taken, and a course of penicillin was begun. The child's course worsened, and he became increasingly lethargic; he developed respiratory distress on the day of admission. It was noted that the throat culture from 3 days prior to admission had not grown any group A streptococci. On examination, the patient was febrile to 38.9°C and had an exudate in the posterior pharynx that was described as a yellowish thick membrane which bled when scraped and removed. The patient's medical history revealed that he had received no immunizations.

1. The patient was admitted to the hospital and treatment was begun. Special cultures of the pharynx were requested that subsequently grew the suspected pathogen. What was this pathogen? Which types of media are used to isolate this organism?

2. To cause disease, does this organism invade the bloodstream? If not, in what way does it cause disease? Which special test is necessary to prove that this organism is capable of producing disease?

3. How can this disease be prevented?

4. How is this disease treated?

DISCUSSION

1. The child appeared to have a strep throat that did not get better. On physical examination, the child had the classic pseudomembrane seen in cases of diphtheria. The etiologic agent of diphtheria is *Corynebacterium diphtheriae,* an aerobic, club-shaped, gram-positive rod. The pseudomembrane seen in patients with diphtheria is composed of bacteria, fibrin, dead epithelial cells, and red and white blood cells. Aspiration of this pseudomembrane can cause death by suffocation.

   It is important that the laboratory be notified when the diagnosis of diphtheria is being considered. Isolation of *C. diphtheriae* is problematic. Throat cultures are not routinely examined for *C. diphtheriae* because the disease is very rare and saprophytic *Corynebacterium* spp., also called diphtheroids, are found in abundance in most throat cultures. These diphtheroids, by both colony and Gram stain morphology, are essentially indistinguishable from *C. diphtheriae.* However, a selective medium, cystine tellurite agar, is useful in the isolation of *C. diphtheriae.* On this medium, *C. diphtheriae* produces black colonies. It should be noted that other diphtheroids and staphylococci will also form similar colonies. Therefore, black colonies must be Gram stained to determine whether they are corynebacteria and then identified biochemically as *C. diphtheriae.* The potassium tellurite salt also suppresses the growth of many organisms which normally inhabit the pharynx.

2. The pathogenesis of *C. diphtheriae* is one of the best understood of any bacteria. The major virulence factor of *C. diphtheriae* is a protein exotoxin called diphtheria toxin. It has been shown to inhibit protein synthesis in a wide variety of mammalian cell types. The gene for toxin production is encoded on a lysogenic phage, and its synthesis is regulated, at least in vitro, by the concentration of iron in the environment of the organism. In patients with diphtheria, the organism remains in the pharynx but the toxin can enter the circulation and inhibit protein synthesis in a variety of tissues, with the heart, nerves, and kidneys being particularly targeted. Both myocarditis and neuropathy can occur in patients with diphtheria.

   Isolates of *C. diphtheriae* which are not lysogenized do not produce diphtheria toxin and are considered nonpathogenic. Since nontoxigenic strains can be isolated from healthy individuals, the isolation of *C. diphtheriae* from the throat alone does not prove that the patient has the disease. Rather, the pathogenic potential of any clinical isolate must be demonstrated by its ability to produce toxin.

3. Vaccination against diphtheria is mandatory in the United States and children are not permitted to attend school without proof of vaccination.

Because the pathogenicity of this organism is due to its exotoxin, a toxoid vaccine has proven to be protective for this disease. Children are given a series of four vaccinations beginning at 2 months of age. They receive the first three doses at approximately 2, 4, and 6 months of age and a booster dose is given 6 to 12 months later. Children receive another booster dose just before entering school. After that, the individuals should receive booster vaccinations at 10-year intervals. Vaccination for diphtheria is given in conjunction with vaccines for *Clostridium tetani* (tetanus) and *Bordetella pertussis* (pertussis). This trivalent vaccine is known as DTP. The 10-year booster doses are composed only of the diphtheria (D) and tetanus (T) component of this vaccine because of the high rate of adverse reactions to the pertussis (P) component.

The vaccination program for eradicating diphtheria in the United States has been highly effective. Usually fewer than 10 cases are reported per year. The cases that do occur are generally in adults, especially among the homeless, who do not receive routine medical care such as booster vaccinations. Cases are also seen in individuals who refuse vaccination for religious reasons.

4. The strategy for treating diphtheria is to use both antibiotics and diphtheria antitoxin. Antitoxin is given to attempt to neutralize circulating diphtheria toxin, since it is responsible for the symptoms caused by this organism. Antibiotics are given to eradicate the organism so that no more toxin can be produced.

The diphtheria antitoxin is prepared in horses, and therefore the development of serum sickness is a distinct possibility. This child was unvaccinated. Because mortality rates of approximately 20% have been reported in unvaccinated individuals, the risk of serum sickness was far outweighed by the potential benefit of giving this antitoxin. Despite appropriate therapy, however, this child died of diphteria.

REFERENCES

Chen, R. T., C. V. Broome, R. A. Weinstein, R. Weaver, and T. F. Tsai. 1985. Diphtheria in the United States. 1971–1981. *Am. J. Public Health* **75:**1393–1397.

Pappenheimer, A. M. 1982. Diphtheria: studies on the biology of an infectious disease. *Harvey Lect.* **76:**45–73.

CASE 10

This 48-year-old man had a long history of alcoholism (including alcoholic hepatitis and hallucinosis) and was admitted to the intensive care unit with profound hypotension and gastrointestinal bleeding. He was intubated and given intravenous fluids and transfused with packed red blood cells (erythrocytes). He remained intubated and ventilator dependent for several weeks. He developed fevers and was treated with broad-spectrum antibiotics. Culture of his tracheal aspirate initially showed *Staphylococcus aureus*. After further antibiotic therapy, Gram stain of his tracheal aspirate showed polymorphonuclear leukocytes and gram-negative rods. His chest radiograph demonstrated an infiltrate and changes consistent with multiple small abscesses. Culture of the tracheal aspirate yielded a heavy growth of an oxidase-positive, beta-hemolytic, gram-negative, lactose-nonfermenting rod that produced a greenish hue on the culture plates. (See Figure 4.)

1. What is the likely agent of infection? Is this organism part of the normal oral flora? Where is it found in the hospital environment? Does it commonly cause pulmonary infections in healthy individuals?

2. This organism produces an exotoxin that is similar to the exotoxin of which other bacteria? How do they act on the host cells?

3. Which pigment(s) does this organism make? What role has been proposed for the pigment(s) in the pathogenicity of this organism?

4. This organism was isolated after the patient received a prolonged course of broad-spectrum antibiotics. Is this organism normally sensitive or resistant to many of the commonly used antibiotics?

5. Bacterial genes may code for a variety of proteins that inactivate antibiotics via a variety of mechanisms. In addition to the bacterial chromosome, where can these genes be found?

DISCUSSION

1. The description of this organism is consistent with *Pseudomonas aeruginosa*. Although certain strains of *Escherichia coli* can be lactose nonfermenting and beta-hemolytic, they are oxidase negative and do not produce pigments. Only *P. aeruginosa* has all the characteristics described in this case.

    During the course of hospitalization, a patient's oropharynx often becomes colonized with both enteric and glucose-nonfermenting gram-negative rods. The exact reason for this colonization is not known.

    The natural habitat of *P. aeruginosa* is water and soil. Raw vegetables, for example, are often contaminated, so foods containing them, such as salads, should be avoided by patients at increased risk for *P. aeruginosa* infections, such as neutropenic patients. Ventilatory equipment often becomes contaminated with *P. aeruginosa* and may act as a source of this agent.

    The organism does not cause pulmonary infections in healthy patients; however, it is the most frequent cause of nosocomial pneumonia, especially in patients receiving ventilatory assistance. It also can chronically infect patients with cystic fibrosis.

2. Over 90% of clinical isolates of *P. aeruginosa* produce an exotoxin designated exotoxin A, which has biological activity similar to that of diphtheria toxin produced by *Corynebacterium diphtheriae*. Both toxins inhibit protein synthesis in eucaryotic cells by catalyzing the transfer of the adenosine diphosphate (ADP)-ribose portion of nicotinamide adenine dinucleotide (NAD) to elongation factor-2 (EF-2). The covalent bonding of this moiety to EF-2 blocks the step in protein synthesis mediated by EF-2, effectively inhibiting it. Interestingly, diphtheria toxin and exotoxin A have biochemically distinct structures and do not show immunologic cross-reactivity. The exact role of exotoxin A in the pathogenesis of *P. aeruginosa* infection of humans is not clear, although this toxin is highly lethal when injected into experimental animals. It is known that this exotoxin is produced in the host since cystic fibrosis patients chronically infected with *P. aeruginosa* have high levels of circulating antibodies to it.

3. This organism may produce four different pigments in various combinations. They are pyoverdin (green), pyocyanin (blue), pyorubin (red), and pyomelanin (brown to black), and their detection is extremely useful in identifying this organism. There has been some preliminary information which suggests that these pigments may act as siderophores (iron-scavenging molecules) for this organism.

4 and 5. One of the reasons why this organism is so effective as a nosocomial pathogen is its resistance to a wide variety of antimicrobial agents. Clini-

cal isolates are routinely resistant to penicillin G, ampicillin, narrow-spectrum and broad-spectrum cephalosporins, chloramphenicol, and trimethoprim-sulfamethoxazole. Most strains also have a chromosomally encoded, inducible β-lactamase. Production of this enzyme is induced by the antimicrobial agents cefoxitin and imipenem. This β-lactamase can degrade the anti-pseudomonal penicillins piperacillin and mezlocillin and the anti-pseudomonal cephalosporin ceftazidime. Its gene appears to undergo mutation at a high rate, especially under antimicrobial pressure, and it can become constitutive as a result of these mutations.

In addition to mutation caused by antimicrobial pressure, this organism may acquire plasmids which code for antimicrobial resistance. Plasmids that code for the production of aminoglycoside-inactivating enzymes are frequently found in *P. aeruginosa*. Antimicrobial pressure appears to be important in maintaining these plasmids. Many of the antimicrobial resistance plasmids may be lost in the absence of this pressure.

REFERENCES

Craven, D. E., and K. A. Steger. 1989. Nosocomial pneumonia in the intubated patient. New concepts on pathogenesis and prevention. *Infect. Dis. Clin. N. Am.* 3:843-866.

Hoiby, N., S. S. Pedersen, G. H. Shand, G. Doring, and I. A. Holder (ed.). 1989. Pseudomonas aeruginosa infection. *Antimicrob. Chemother.* 42:1-300.

The patient was a 34-year-old male with a history of tobacco and alcohol abuse (12 cans of beer per day). Two months prior to admission he was seen at an outside hospital, where he was found to have a necrotic lesion in his right upper lobe. He was PPD (purified protein derivative) negative and three sputum cultures done for *Mycobacterium* spp. were negative. He had no risk factors for human immunodeficiency virus (HIV) infection. Four weeks prior to admission, he presented with fever, productive cough, night sweats, chills, and a 10-lb (4.5-kg) weight loss. He was treated with ampicillin-clavulanic acid for 14 days. Fever, chills, and night sweats decreased. On admission, he presented with a firm right chest wall mass (4 by 4 cm), which was aspirated. The aspirated material was dark green and extremely viscous. Two days later, the nurses found him urinating on the wall of his room. Because this was unusual behavior for this patient, it was decided to perform a computed tomogram (CT scan) of the head; the scan revealed multiple, ring-enhancing lesions. The patient was taken to surgery and the central nervous system (CNS) lesions were drained. A Gram stain of the organism recovered from the brain aspirate showed a branching, beaded gram-positive rod. (See Figure 5.)

1. What do the lesions in the patient's head probably indicate? What therapy does this patient need?

2. Explain the relationship between his chest wall lesion and his brain lesions.

3. Which lifestyle factor(s) predisposed this patient to the chest wall lesion?

4. What is the origin of the organism causing this patient's infection?

5. Two genera of organisms are likely on the basis of the Gram stain. Which test could be performed on the brain aspirate to determine the genus to which this organism belonged?

DISCUSSION

1. Ring-enhancing lesions in the brain usually are associated with infection. The appropriate therapy for this patient would be to drain the CNS lesions, probably by aspiration, and then start appropriate antimicrobial therapy. This manuever has both therapeutic and diagnostic value. Abscesses are rarely cured by antimicrobial therapy alone, but also require drainage. The reason for this is that antimicrobial agents probably will not penetrate to the center of these purulent lesions at high enough levels to kill or inhibit the growth of the infecting organism(s). By determining the exact etiology of the infection, the most appropriate antimicrobial therapy can be used.

2. Brain abscesses are seen in limited clinical settings, usually as secondary infections in patients with lung abscesses (such as in this patient), endocarditis, sinusitis, head trauma, and meningitis. Both in endocarditis and in lung abscesses, septic emboli (small blood clots contaminated with microorganisms) break away from the lesion and enter the circulation. These emboli can enter the circulation of the brain and actually block the capillary bed in the brain tissue. This blockage results in hemorrhage and local infection, which can develop into an abscess.

3 and 4. Excessive alcohol consumption can result in unconscious states. Clearance of oral secretions is believed to be depressed as a result of a decreased gag reflex and/or the alcohol-induced stupor. As a result, members of the oropharyngeal flora, which are usually easily cleared, can infect the lower airways. In addition, vomiting can lead to aspiration of gastric acid and enzymes, which can cause localized tissue damage and create an ideal focus for infection. The end result can be a lung abscess followed by a secondary brain abscess.

5. Organisms which on Gram stain appear as branching, beaded gram-positive rods and frequently cause infection are limited to two genera, *Actinomyces* and *Nocardia* spp. They can be differentiated by a modified acid-fast stain. *Nocardia* spp. are partially acid fast, whereas *Actinomyces* spp. are not. In addition, *Nocardia* spp. are strict aerobes, whereas *Actinomyces* spp. prefer anaerobic growth conditions.

   It is important to differentiate these organisms because therapy for them is different. This patient's specimen grew *Actinomyces* spp. from both chest wall and brain aspirates. A modified acid-fast stain done on the material aspirated from the brain was negative.

REFERENCE

Wispelwey, B., and W. M. Scheld. 1990. Brain abscess, p. 777–786. *In* G. L. Mandell, R. G. Douglas, Jr., and J. E. Bennett (ed.), *Principles and Practice of Infectious Diseases*, 3rd ed. Churchill Livingstone Inc., New York.

The patient was a 55-year-old male with a 2-month history of fevers, night sweats, increased cough with sputum production, and a 25-lb (ca. 11-kg) weight loss. The patient denied intravenous (i.v.) drug use or homosexual activity. He has had multiple sexual encounters, "sips" a pint of gin a day, was jailed 2 years ago in New York City, and has a history of gunshot and stab wounds. His physical examination was significant for bilateral anterior cervical and axillary adenopathy and a temperature of 39.4°C. His chest radiograph showed paratracheal adenopathy and bilateral interstitial infiltrates. His laboratory findings were significant for a positive HIV serology and a low absolute CD4$^+$ lymphocyte count. An acid-fast organism grew from the sputum and bronchoalveolar lavage fluid from the right middle lobe.

1. What is bronchoalveolar lavage fluid? How is it obtained? What is its value as a diagnostic specimen?

2. Which organisms can be positive on an acid-fast stain?

3. Given his medical history, which organism is this likely to be? How does the finding that the patient is HIV positive affect this decision?

4. Which factors in his medical history do you think are important in his contracting this infection with acid-fast bacteria?

5. What is a PPD test? What is its value in this patient? What additional tests would you order with a PPD test?

DISCUSSION

1. Bronchoalveolar lavage is performed during bronchoscopy. The broncho-scope is wedged into the bronchus of the lobe in which disease is seen by radiographic examination or by visual inspection of the airway. Approximately 100 to 200 ml of nonbacteriostatic saline is injected through a channel in the bronchoscope into a specific lobe. This large volume of saline lavages the alveoli. The lavage fluid containing inflammatory cells and, in cases of infection, infectious agents is aspirated from the lung through the bronchoscope. This method is particularly useful in recovering viral agents and detecting *Pneumocystis carinii*. This is a very effective way of collecting contents of the alveoli of the lung without these contents being contaminated with organisms from the upper airways (as would be seen with sputum). In patients without cough or with nonproductive cough, bronchoscopy is the simplest way to adequately sample the lungs.

2. The most important organisms which are acid fast are mycobacteria. Other organisms of clinical importance which are either completely or partially acid fast include *Rhodococcus equi, Nocardia* spp., and the protozoans *Cryptosporidium* spp. and *Isospora* spp.

3. The most likely organism is *Mycobacterium tuberculosis*. The finding that the individual is HIV positive should not alter this decision. Being HIV positive is now recognized as an important risk factor for the development of tuberculosis. In fact, tuberculosis in HIV-infected individuals has been cited as a major reason for the reversal in a long-term trend of a steady decline in the number of cases of tuberculosis in the United States. This trend is particularly striking in HIV-infected intravenous drug users. One issue that has become a particular public health concern is the increasing numbers of *M. tuberculosis* isolates that are being recovered from AIDS patients that are resistant to the first-line anti-tuberculous drugs isoniazid and rifampin. Spread of multi-drug-resistant organisms from this patient population to their caregivers has been reported. Also frequently seen in HIV-positive individuals are organisms of the *Mycobacterium avium* complex. These organisms are particularly problematic in HIV-infected patients because anti-tuberculous antimicrobial therapy is ineffective against them, as is the immune system of these individuals.

4. Factors which put him at increased risk for tuberculosis (TB) are his HIV seropositivity, his alcoholism, and the fact that he had recently been jailed. This disease is more prevalent in individuals with any one of these risk factors. The presence of all three risk factors only increases the likelihood of his having TB. His clinical presentation is also typical for tuberculosis except that apical regions of the lung are the most commonly affected in

active disease. Cavitary lesions, which are frequently seen in normal hosts, are unusual in HIV-infected patients. This may reflect their immunocompromised state and inability to develop cell-mediated immune responses to the mycobacterial infection.

5. A PPD test is a skin test used to screen individuals for *M. tuberculosis* infection. PPD is a *M. tuberculosis* antigen that is injected intracutaneously on the forearm with a tuberculin syringe. The forearm is examined at the site of injection 48 and 72 h later. In HIV-seronegative individuals who have no known close contact with tuberculosis-infected patients, an area of induration of 10 mm indicates a positive PPD test; these individuals should receive preventive tuberculosis therapy. It should be noted that most PPD-positive patients are asymptomatically infected. The immunosuppression which occurs as a result of HIV infection may lead to false-negative skin tests. When testing an HIV-positive patient, a concurrent control skin test for anergy (usually done using a candidal or tetanus toxoid antigen) should be done to determine whether the patient is even capable of reacting to common antigens. Negative PPD tests are uninterpretable in anergic individuals. An area of induration of ≥ 5 mm in an HIV-seropositive individual is sufficient to require therapy, but more definitive evidence of infection, such as a positive chest radiograph, should be sought.

REFERENCES

Centers for Disease Control. 1990. Update: tuberculosis elimination—United States. *Morbid. Mortal. Weekly Rep.* **39:**153–156.

Centers for Disease Control. 1990. Screening for tuberculosis and tuberculosis infection in high-risk populations and the use of preventive therapy for tuberculous infections in the United States. *Morbid. Mortal. Weekly. Rep.* **39 (RR-8):**1–12.

Selwyn, P. A., D. Hartel, V. A. Lewis, E. E. Schoenbaum, S. H. Vermund, R. S. Klein, A. T. Walker, and G. H. Friedland. 1989. A prospective study of the risk of tuberculosis among intravenous drug users with human immunodeficiency virus infection. *N. Engl. J. Med.* **320:**545–550.

This 40-year-old male was transferred to our hospital via helicopter with multisystem failure secondary to bilateral pneumonia. He had presented to his local physician 3 days previously complaining of fevers, malaise, and vague respiratory symptoms. He was given amantadine for suspected influenza. His condition became progressively worse and he developed shortness of breath and a fever to 40.5°C and was admitted to an outside hospital 24 h prior to transfer. A laboratory examination revealed abnormal liver and renal function. Therapy with Timentin (ticarcillin-clavulanic acid) and trimethoprim-sulfamethoxazole was begun. On admission, he underwent a bronchoscopic examination which revealed mildly inflamed airways containing thin, watery secretions. A Gram stain of bronchial washings obtained at bronchoscopy revealed a few polymorphonuclear cells and alveolar macrophages and few, poorly staining gram-negative rods. Based on these findings, he was begun on appropriate antimicrobial therapy. Culture results were positive for a gram-negative rod which grew on a medium specially designed to support its growth but failed to grow on chocolate agar. Nine months later this patient died after being moved to a long-term care facility.

1. Which organisms are common causes of community-acquired bacterial pneumonia?

2. What are bronchial washings and how are they obtained?

3. On the basis of the Gram stain of the bronchial washings and the patient's presentation, what is the most likely cause of this patient's catastrophic infection? Why must the laboratory be notified if this organism is considered in the differential diagnosis?

4. How can the definitive diagnosis of this infection be made rapidly?

5. What is the epidemiology of this organism?

6. What is the appropriate antimicrobial agent for treatment of this infection? Which other gram-negative respiratory pathogen is treated with this agent?

DISCUSSION

1. The common causes of community-acquired pneumonia are *Streptococcus pneumoniae*; *Haemophilus influenzae*; *Mycoplasma pneumoniae*; *Staphylococcus aureus*, frequently secondary to influenza virus; *Klebsiella pneumoniae*, especially in the elderly and alcoholics; and *Legionella pneumophila*.

2. Bronchial washings are obtained during bronchoscopic examination. The bronchoscope is introduced, and a small volume of saline is injected into the bronchi through a channel in the bronchoscope. The saline/bronchial secretions mixture is then suctioned from the bronchi through the bronchoscope and is sent to the laboratory for staining and culture.

3. This patient had *L. pneumophila* pneumonia. *L. pneumophila* is an aerobic, poorly staining gram-negative rod. Legionellae are fastidious organisms and will not grow on media routinely used for cultivation of respiratory secretions. The laboratory must be notified so that a special medium, buffered charcoal yeast extract agar (BCYE), which will support the growth of this organism, is used.

    This case demonstrates the catastrophic nature of this illness in some previously healthy patients. Key findings in this case include hepatic and renal dysfunction, as well as the finding of thin, watery secretions, which are characteristics of pneumonia with this infection. Patients with bacterial pneumonia due to other agents generally have thick, purulent secretions.

4. *L. pneumophila* can be rapidly detected in three ways: by performing a direct fluorescent antibody (DFA) test, by using a gene probe, or by detecting *Legionella* antigen in urine. All three tests have been used in clinical settings. The DFA test and gene probe have a sensitivity when compared with culture of 60 to 70%; i.e., 3 or 4 of 10 patients culture positive for *L. pneumophila* will not be detected by these tests. However, these tests take only 2 h, compared with up to 5 days for culture to become positive, so they are useful. The urine antigen detection test is more sensitive than the other two tests but is not widely used because it requires the use of a radioisotope.

5. *L. pneumophila* was first recognized as a cause of pneumonia when an outbreak of pneumonia of unknown etiology called Legionnaires disease occurred in 1976 during an American Legion convention in Philadelphia. The organism was traced to the air-conditioning system at one of the convention hotels. Exposure to water containing *L. pneumophila* is believed to be its major mode of transmission. There is no evidence of person-to-person transmission. A number of studies have shown *L. pneu-*

mophila to be the etiologic agent in nosocomial outbreaks of pneumonia. A common theme in all of these outbreaks was the aerosolization of water contaminated with *L. pneumophila*. The organism grows in air-conditioning systems, shower heads, tap water, and sinks. It is very difficult to eradicate from hospital water supplies, although superheating and hyperchlorination of water have both been used with various degrees of success. Despite concern about nosocomial outbreaks of *L. pneumophila* infection, sporadic community-acquired cases are probably more common in the United States. Chronic lung disease, immunosuppression, and advancing age all have been implicated as risk factors. Our patient had none of these. A possible risk factor in this patient may have been viral pneumonia prior to his *Legionella* infection. Although prior viral infection is not recognized as a risk factor for *L. pneumophila* pneumonia, it is well recognized that bacterial superinfection can follow viral pneumonia, and this patient's original presentation may have been due to a virus such as influenza virus. Alternatively, *L. pneumophila* can cause a "flu-like" prodrome, and all his symptoms may be explained by his *L. pneumophila* infection.

6. Erythromycin is the therapy of choice. This agent is usually considered to be active only against gram-positive organisms. However, it is known to be active against two gram-negative rods which cause infection in the respiratory tract, *Legionella* spp. and *Bordetella pertussis*. A key characteristic of this antimicrobial agent is its ability to penetrate into white cells. This characteristic is probably important therapeutically since *Legionella* spp. can survive and multiply within macrophages. Beta-lactam drugs have proven to be ineffective against *L. pneumophila* due in part to its ability to produce a beta-lactamase.

REFERENCES

Edelstein, P. H., R. N. Bryan, R. K. Enns, D. E. Kohne, and D. L. Kacian. 1987. Retrospective study of Gen-Probe rapid diagnostic system for detection of legionellae in frozen clinical respiratory tract specimens. *J. Clin. Microbiol.* **25:**1022–1026.

Fraser, D. W., T. R. Tsai, W. Orenstein, W. E. Parkin, H. J. Beecham, R. G. Sharrar, J. Harris, G. F. Mallison, S. M. Martin, J. E. McDade, C. C. Shepard, P. S. Brachman, and The Field Investigation Team. 1977. Legionnaires' disease. Description of an epidemic of pneumonia. *N. Engl. J. Med.* **297:**1189–1203.

Ruf, B., D. Shurmann, I. Horbach, F. J. Fehrenbach, and H. D. Pohle. 1990. Prevalence and diagnosis of *Legionella* pneumonia: a 3-year prospective study with emphasis on application of urinary antigen detection. *J. Infect. Dis.* **162:**1341–1348.

The patient was a 32-year-old Haitian male referred to the hospital with a 3-week history of fever, nausea, vomiting, and diarrhea. Four days after returning from Haiti, where he had seen unembalmed bodies at a funeral, he developed a temperature to 39.5°C, myalgias, constipation, and rectal pain. He was admitted to an outside hospital overnight and given i.v. cefotaxime. He was discharged on oral cephalexin. His symptoms recurred 1 week prior to admission, and his therapy was changed to metronidazole. Five days prior to admission, the patient developed fever, diarrhea with six watery stools per day, nausea, vomiting, and dark urine. On the day of admission, the patient passed out while walking to the bathroom.

On admission, he had a temperature of 37.7°C, supine pulse rate of 104 beats/min and blood pressure of 115/75 mmHg; the standing pulse rate and blood pressure were 132 beats/min and 90/60 mmHg, respectively. The rest of the patient's physical and laboratory findings were unremarkable. On the second hospital day, the patient became acutely agitated, pulled out his i.v. lines, and tried to leave the hospital. He claimed that a voodoo curse had been placed on him and that he was "already dead." Hepatitis and HIV serologic tests were negative. Blood and stool cultures were diagnostic.

1. Explain the significance of the patient's travel history.

2. Why did the patient pass out on his way to the bathroom? Would his vital signs on admission explain why he passed out?

3. Organisms were found in both blood and stool. Briefly explain the pathogenesis of the bacteremia.

4. Which other types of clinical specimens might be useful for culture in this disease?

5. What was the etiologic agent of infection?

6. If this person worked in the food industry, what action should be taken before he was allowed to return to work?

DISCUSSION

1. In patients with febrile illnesses, a travel history can often be helpful, especially if patients have been to areas which have infectious agents not found in the United States (malaria, yellow fever, etc.). Individuals who travel to developing countries such as Haiti, with poor sanitation which can result in fecal contamination of water and food, are at increased risk for infections acquired by the fecal-oral route, such as typhoid fever.

2. Because of a 5-day history of diarrhea and vomiting, it is likely that the patient was dehydrated. Dehydration leads to depletion in intravascular volume. This decrease in volume results in postural (supine versus standing) changes in heart rate and blood pressure. When this patient stood to go to the bathroom, his blood pressure dropped, causing him to pass out.

3. The organism is spread by ingestion of fecally contaminated food or water. A fairly high inoculum (10^6 organisms) is needed because these organisms are rapidly killed at pH 2, the pH of the normal stomach. The organisms which survive their transit through the stomach then multiply in the small intestine. They attach to microvilli in the ileum and jejunum and penetrate the intestinal mucosa. They are transported to Peyer's patches, where they can multiply within macrophages. From the Peyer's patches, they can be carried to the bloodstream via the lymphatics.

4. Bone marrow culture is the specimen of choice in making the diagnosis of typhoid fever when routine blood and stool cultures are negative. Bone marrow cultures are positive in approximately 90% of patients. Conventional blood cultures are positive in only 50% of patients, and stool cultures are positive in only 33%. Some textbooks advocate urine cultures, but they are rarely positive (<10%).

5. The infectious agent was *Salmonella typhi*. The organism is an enteric lactose-nonfermenting gram-negative rod. A key biochemical characteristic of *S. typhi* is its ability to produce a small ring of H_2S on triple sugar iron agar slants at the top of the butt. Other *Salmonella* isolates will produce H_2S throughout the butt.

6. Approximately 1 to 3% of patients who have typhoid fever will become chronic carriers of *S. typhi*. They excrete large numbers (10^6 CFU/ml) of *S. typhi* cells in their feces and can continue to do so for many years. Food workers who do not practice good hygiene could contaminate the food they handle, spreading the organisms to large numbers of individuals. As a result, workers in the food industry should have three negative stool cultures for *S. typhi* before being allowed to return to work. These cultures

should be done over a period of at least 5 to 7 days to prevent sampling error.

In the carrier state, the organisms reside in the biliary tree and are excreted in bile. We recently saw a 80-year-old patient who had just had his gallbladder removed. He gave his surgeon a history of having had typhoid fever when he was 20 but excellent health since then. The surgeon sent a swab of the patient's gallbladder for culture, and it grew *S. typhi* 60 years after his original infection!

REFERENCES

Gilman, R. H., M. Terminel, M. M. Levine, P. Hernandez-Mendoza, and R. B. Hornick. 1975. Relative efficacy of blood, urine, bone-marrow, and ros-spot cultures for recovery of *Salmonella typhi* in typhoid fever. *Lancet* i:1211–1213.

Taylor, D. N., R. A. Pollard, and P. A. Blake. 1983. Typhoid in the United States and the risk to the international traveler. *J. Infect. Dis.* 148:599–602.

This 18-year-old male presented to the outpatient medical clinic for evaluation of diarrhea and abdominal discomfort. The patient first noted mild abdominal discomfort and three loose bowel movements per day 1 week prior to evaluation. Two days prior to evaluation he noted intermittent, crampy periumbilical abdominal pain. He denied fever, blood in the stool, relation of the pain to meals, drinking well water, dysuria, or hematuria.

On examination, the patient was afebrile and had normal vital signs. The abdominal examination was notable for mild lower abdominal tenderness. The fecal examination demonstrated a greenish, watery stool that was negative for occult blood.

Laboratory evaluation included a normal white blood cell count, hematocrit, and platelet count. Examination of the feces microscopically was remarkable for the presence of white blood cells. The causative agent recovered from feces was a slightly curved, gram-negative rod.

1. On the basis of the laboratory findings, what is the likely etiology of this patient's diarrhea? Are the finding of white cells in his feces consistent with the recovery of this organism? Explain your answer.

2. What special laboratory conditions are necessary to recover this organism?

3. What is the epidemiology of this organism? What interventions can prevent its spread?

4. Although the patient has evidence of local invasion in the intestinal tract with this organism, bacteremia due to this organism is unusual. Explain this observation.

DISCUSSION

1. Both *Vibrio* and *Campylobacter* spp. are slightly curved, gram-negative rods that cause diarrhea. The pathogenesis of the most important *Vibrio* species, *Vibrio cholerae,* is due primarily to the production of an exotoxin, cholera toxin, which causes a secretory diarrhea. The stools of patients with severe cases of cholera have a "rice water" appearance. Because of the secretory, noninflammatory nature of the diarrhea, white blood cells are rarely seen in the feces of patients with cholera. *Campylobacter* spp. cause an invasive diarrhea manifested by the presence of white blood cells in the stool. The diarrhea seen in this patient is consistent with a *Campylobacter* sp., and *Campylobacter jejuni* was isolated from his stool.

2. It is important to remember that the aerobic fecal flora consists of approximately 10^7 to 10^9 CFU/g of feces and that finding an enteric pathogen which may represent only a small fraction of this flora is akin to trying to find a needle in a haystack. Selective media, such as Hektoen and MacConkey agar, used for the isolation of *Salmonella* and *Shigella* spp. from feces, do not support the growth of *Campylobacter* spp. Therefore several selective media have been developed for the isolation of *Campylobacter* spp. To further complicate matters, *Campylobacter* spp. are microaerophilic organisms, and so culture conditions which will support their growth must be used when attempting to isolate them. Finally, *C. jejuni,* the most frequently recovered *Campylobacter* species, grows optimally at 42°C. Many laboratories inoculate fecal specimens onto campylobacter selective agar and incubate these plates at 42°C under microaerophilic conditions in an attempt to isolate these organisms. This approach is problematic since other *Campylobacter* spp. either fail to grow on certain types of campylobacter selective agar or cannot grow at 42°C. Alternative methods are available for the isolation of these species.

3. *C. jejuni,* like all enteric pathogens, is spread by the fecal-oral route. It is frequently recovered from poultry carcasses. Improperly cooked poultry or cross-contamination of foods by raw poultry is postulated to be the most important source of infection. Outbreaks of *Campylobacter* infection have also followed the consumption of nonpasteurized milk. Contaminated water is an infrequent vehicle for this infection. Adequate cooking of poultry and avoidance of cross-contamination of other foods will result in prevention of most *Campylobacter* cases. The infectious dose for this organism appears to be intermediate between those for *Shigella* spp. (low) and *Salmonella* spp. (high). Like *Salmonella* and *Shigella,* it is an organism which causes disease mainly during the warm-weather months. One of the interesting observations concerning this organism is that the peak

incidence of infection is in infants (<1 year old) and adolescents and young adults (15 to 29 years old). It is probably the most frequent cause of bacterial gastroenteritis in college students, with isolation rates on certain campuses as high as 15%.

4. *C. jejuni* was locally invasive in this patient as evidenced by the presence of white blood cells in his feces. Like *Shigella* spp., this organism rarely causes bacteremia in the immunocompetent host. The most likely reason for this is that this organism, unlike *Salmonella* spp., does not survive within phagocytic cells. It is either locally ingested and killed by phagocytes in the intestinal wall or carried by lymphatic drainage to the Peyer's patches, where it is killed. Occasional cases of *C. jejuni* bacteremia occur, but most are transient because the reticuloendothelial system is able to eliminate this organism from the bloodstream.

REFERENCES

Cornick, N. A., and S. L. Gorbach. 1988. Campylobacter. *Infect. Dis. Clin. N. Am.* **2:**643–654.

Finch, M. J., and L. W. Riley. 1984. Campylobacter infections in the United States. *Arch. Intern. Med.* **144:**1610–1612.

This 30-year-old dairy farmer was in good health until the day prior to admission, when he felt chilled and feverish. He developed nausea, vomiting, diarrhea, and lower abdominal discomfort and presented to the emergency room, where he was noted to be lethargic. His vital signs included temperature of 40°C, blood pressure of 100/60 mmHg in the supine position and 80/60 mmHg sitting, and a pulse of 80 beats/min. His physical examination was remarkable for lower abdominal tenderness to palpation bilaterally. A rectal examination revealed occult blood in the stool. The patient was lethargic but had no focal neurological deficits. Of note, his 3-year-old child had been discharged from the hospital 2 days previously with a similar history.

The patient underwent a lumbar puncture because of his altered mental status and fever. Laboratory studies of cerebrospinal fluid (CSF) were within normal limits, and a bacterial culture of CSF was negative.

The patient was treated with i.v. fluids and antibiotics, and his condition improved. A stool examination for fecal leukocytes was positive, and a stool culture was diagnostic. Biochemical examination of the organism revealed it to be a lactose nonfermenter on MacConkey agar, H_2S negative, urea negative, and nonmotile at both 25 and 37°C.

1. Which organisms would be in your differential diagnosis of bloody diarrhea with fecal leukocytes?

2. On the basis of the biochemical reactions, which organism do you think this is?

3. What are the antimicrobial agents of choice to treat this infection? Should they be used in this clinical setting?

4. Did this person have meningitis? Explain your answer.

5. How is dehydration in patients with diarrhea usually treated? Why could this therapy not be used in this case?

6. This patient's wife and another child also had this infection. Was this individual's vocation, dairy farming, important in the epidemiology of this infection in his family? Explain your answer.

DISCUSSION

1. The presence of fecal leukocytes is indicative of inflammatory diarrhea due to an invasive enteropathogen. In developing our differential diagnosis, we will concentrate on bacterial agents, although protozoans also may cause an inflammatory diarrhea.

   The bacterial agents most likely to cause inflammatory diarrhea are *Salmonella* spp., *Shigella* spp., *Campylobacter* spp., *Yersinia* spp., and enteroinvasive *Escherichia coli* (note: these strains of *E. coli* contain genes for *Shigella*-derived virulence factors). Bloody diarrhea can also be caused by *E. coli* isolates which produce verotoxin. These isolates are called enterohemorrhagic *E. coli*. Our experience is that white cells are frequently present in the feces of patients infected with this agent. The verotoxin, which is believed to be responsible for pathophysiological changes associated with this organism, is biochemically and immunologically very similar to Shiga toxin produced by *Shigella dysenteriae* and has also been referred to in the scientific literature as "Shiga-like toxin."

2. From the biochemical reactions of this organism, it is most likely to be a *Shigella* sp. Its ability to grow on MacConkey agar eliminates *Campylobacter* spp. from consideration. Its inability to produce H_2S and its lack of motility eliminate *Salmonella* spp. Since the organism is nonmotile at 25°C and is urea negative, *Yersinia* spp. are eliminated.

3. Ampicillin is the drug of choice for treatment of shigellosis. If ampicillin resistance is detected or is endemic, trimethoprim-sulfamethoxazole can also be used. Concurrent resistance to both these agents is very unusual in the United States. Adults can also be treated with tetracycline and ciprofloxacin, which are not used in children. Because of the severity of his illness, antimicrobial therapy is important in this patient. It should be emphasized that the use of antimicrobial agents to treat mild cases of shigellosis is controversial. The benefit is that they decrease the length of shedding of the organism. Because *Shigella* spp. are spread from person to person usually via a vehicle such as food or water, and the infectious dose is quite small (<10 organisms), decreased shedding should result in decreased spread. This is particularly important in settings such as day-care centers where outbreaks of shigellosis are frequent. However, there is a risk of increased antimicrobial resistance which may follow antimicrobial therapy. In patients who are not in potential contact with large numbers of people and have mild disease, antimicrobial therapy may not be warranted.

4. Because his cerebrospinal fluid examination was normal, this individual did not have meningitis. His central nervous system symptoms may have

been secondary to either dehydration or the activity of Shiga toxin, a known neurotoxin. Dehydration, as evidenced by his low blood pressure, may cause electrolyte imbalances and hence altered mental status.

5. One of the major advances in the fight against diarrheal disease, a killer of 5 million people worldwide each year, is oral rehydration therapy. Oral rehydration fluid is a simple mixture of glucose and electrolytes which is inexpensive and easy to administer. Glucose stimulates the uptake of electrolytes by the intestinal epithelium, with water passing across the intestinal epithelium osmotically. In this case the patient was vomiting and so oral rehydration therapy and oral antibiotics would probably have failed.

6. Dairy farmers are at increased risk for diarrheal disease caused by *Salmonella* spp., various enteropathogenic *E. coli* isolates, and *Campylobacter* spp., all of which can infect dairy cattle. Since humans are the primary hosts of *Shigella* spp., this organism does not infect cattle; therefore, his vocation played no role in the spread of infection. It was speculated either that this family's well water was contaminated or that the food they had eaten during a family reunion picnic recently held at the home was the source of their infection. Other family members who attended the picnic also developed shigellosis.

REFERENCE

DuPont, H. L. 1988. Shigella. *Infect. Dis. Clin. N. Am.* **2:**599–606.

CASE **17**

The patient was a 37-year-old male with hemophilia. He was HIV positive and had progressed from AIDS-related complex (ARC) to AIDS in the past 3 months. He had a number of previous admissions, the most recent for *Pneumocystis carinii* pneumonia. His current therapeutic regimen included factor VIII treatments, suppressive trimethoprim-sulfamethoxazole, and azidothymidine (AZT). He presented with a 3-day history of voluminous diarrhea, 10-lb (ca. 4.5-kg) weight loss, and profound dehydration. Methylene blue stain of stool was negative for white cells. An examination for occult blood was also negative. Tests for ova and parasites and culture for *Salmonella, Shigella, Yersinia,* and *Campylobacter* spp. were negative three times. He gave no recent travel history, nor had he recently consumed shellfish.

1. Which types of enteric pathogens are usually ruled out by a negative examination for fecal leukocytes and occult blood?

2. Why was it important to elicit a travel history from this individual?

3. What role do suppressive antimicrobial agents have in predisposing this patient to his current infection?

4. What was the etiologic agent of infection in this patient? How is the microbiological diagnosis of this agent best made?

5. Why is it important to establish an etiology for diarrhea in this patient?

DISCUSSION

1. Methylene blue stain for fecal leukocytes and examination for occult blood are usually positive when invasive diarrhea is due to *Salmonella* spp., *Shigella* spp., enteroinvasive *E. coli, Yersinia enterocolitica,* or *Campylobacter* spp. A negative stain and examination for occult blood indicate a noninflammatory diarrhea, and hence the agents of invasive diarrhea are much less likely.

2. The type of diarrhea described in this case is consistent with enterotoxigenic *E. coli* or *Vibrio cholerae.* These organisms are endemic only in limited regions of the country, and this patient did not live in an endemic region. It would be highly unusual for him to be infected with either organism without a history of travel to an area of endemicity, or a history of consumption of shellfish, either raw or improperly cooked. Shellfish are filter feeders and when living in waters containing *V. cholerae,* they may become contaminated with this organism.

3. Antimicrobial therapy alters the bowel flora. Infectious doses of enteric pathogens such as *Salmonella* spp. are probably lowered as a result. This lowering of the infectious dose is probably due to decreased competition for binding sites on the epithelium of the bowel. *Clostridium difficile* is a frequent cause of antibiotic-associated diarrhea and enterocolitis. In *C. difficile* disease, the situation is slightly different from that seen with *Salmonella* spp. *C. difficile* may be part of the normal flora in some individuals. The number of *C. difficile* organisms in the bowel is probably small in these individuals because components of the normal bowel flora can suppress the growth of *C. difficile.* When the normal bowel flora is disrupted and the *C. difficile*-inhibitory flora is reduced or eliminated, *C. difficile* can grow and begin to produce two different exotoxins. These exotoxins are responsible for the pathophysiological changes seen in this disease.

4. The patient was suffering from *C. difficile* enterocolitis. The laboratory diagnosis of this infection is made by direct detection of one of the two *C. difficile* exotoxins in the stool. The two toxins are cytotoxin and enterotoxin. Cytotoxin is best detected by applying fecal filtrates to tissue culture monolayers. The cells are observed for cytopathic effects characterized by a rounding of the cells over 48 h. If cytopathic effects are seen, antiserum against *C. difficile* is mixed with cytopathic fecal filtrates, applied to monolayers, and observed for neutralization of the cytopathic effect. Nonimmune serum is also mixed with an aliquot of the same fecal filtrate as a positive control.

Enterotoxin can be detected by using an enzyme immunosorbent assay (EIA). It is more rapid than the cytotoxicity assay but is somewhat less sensitive.

Culture is not useful in making this diagnosis for two reasons. First, approximately 20% of patients on antibiotics who do not have diarrhea harbor this organism. Second, a significant percentage of *C. difficile* isolates are nontoxigenic and thus are unable to cause disease.

5. Many causes of diarrheal diseases in AIDS patients, e.g., *Cryptosporidium* and *Microsporidium* spp., are untreatable, and this may contribute to premature death. *C. difficile* is treatable with either oral vancomycin or metronidazole. This patient recovered with appropriate therapy and had many more productive months of life.

REFERENCES

Bartlett, J. G. 1979. Antibiotic-associated pseudomembraneous colitis. *Rev. Infect. Dis.* 1:530–539.

Lyerly, D. M., H. C. Krivan, and T. D. Wilkins. 1988. *Clostridum difficile*: its disease and toxins. *Clin. Microbiol. Rev.* 1:1–18.

The patient was a 19-year-old female with a history of a urinary tract infection (UTI) 4 months prior to admission for which she was treated with oral ampicillin without complications. Five days prior to this admission she began to note nausea without vomiting. One day later she developed left flank pain, fevers, and chills and noted increased urinary frequency. She noted foul-smelling urine on the day prior to admission. She presented with a temperature of 38.8°C, and physical examination showed left costovertebral angle tenderness. Urinalysis of a clean-catch urine sample was notable for >50 white blood cells per high-power field, 3 to 10 red blood cells per high-power field, and 3+ bacteria. Urine culture was subsequently positive for >100,000 CFU of a gram-negative, lactose-fermenting rod per ml (see Figure 6); this bacterium was beta-hemolytic on sheep blood agar.

1. What do the urinalysis findings indicate? Explain your answer.

2. Why were the numbers of organisms in her urine quantitated on culture? How would you interpret the culture results in this case?

3. Which gram-negative rods are lactose fermenters? Which ones are also beta-hemolytic?

4. The urinary isolate was spot indole positive. How does this information help in its identification?

5. This bacterium was resistant to ampicillin. What in this patient's history might explain this observation?

6. Urinary tract infections are more frequent in women than men. Why?

7. Did this woman have cystitis or pyelonephritis? Why is it important to differentiate the two?

DISCUSSION

1. Urine from normal individuals usually has fewer than 10 white blood cells per high-power field. Pyuria (the presence of >10 white blood cells per high-power field in urine) and hematuria (the presence of red blood cells in urine), as seen in this patient, are reasonably sensitive although not always specific indicators of urinary tract infection. The presence of bacteriuria (bacteria in urine) in this patient further supports this diagnosis. However, the presence of bacteriuria on urinalysis should always be interpreted with caution. Clean-catch urine is rarely sterile because the distal urethra is colonized with bacteria. Urine is an excellent growth medium. Therefore, if urine is not analyzed fairly quickly (within 1 h), the organisms colonizing the urethra can divide (2 to 3 generations per h) and may be present in sufficient numbers to be visualized during urinalysis even though the patient is not infected.

2. In a normal individual, urine within the bladder is sterile. As it passes through the urethra, which has a resident microflora, it almost always becomes contaminated with a small number ($<10^3$ CFU/ml) of organisms. Clean-catch urine samples are obtained when midstream urine is voided directly into a collecting device, usually a sterile cup, after the external genitalia have been cleansed. As a result of urethral contamination, essentially all clean catch urine samples will contain a small number of organisms, so culturing urine nonquantitatively will not allow differentiation between colonization of the urethra and infection of the bladder.

   Patients in whom the bladder is infected tend to have very large numbers of bacteria in their urine. These organisms usually, but not always, are of a single species. Studies have shown that most individuals with true urinary tract infections have greater than 100,000 CFU/ml in clean-catch urine specimens. There are exceptions to this generalization, but discussion of them is beyond the scope of this book. (The interested student can read references 2 and 3 for further information on this topic.) The patient's clinical presentation and culture results of >100,000 CFU/ml indicate that she has a urinary tract infection.

3. The lactose fermenters that are most commonly isolated from urine are the KEE organisms (i.e., *Klebsiella* spp., *Escherichia coli*, and *Enterobacter* spp.) *E. coli* is recovered from approximately 70 to 80% of outpatients and 40 to 50% of inpatients with urinary tract infections. The observation that the organism is beta-hemolytic indicates that, in all likelihood, the organism is *E. coli*. Approximately 60% of *E. coli* isolates recovered from urine are reported to be beta-hemolytic, whereas *Klebsiella* and *Enterobacter* spp. are rarely, if ever, beta-hemolytic. Another common gram-negative rod which

is frequently beta-hemolytic is *Pseudomonas aeruginosa*. It is incapable of fermenting carbohydrates and should not be confused with lactose-fermenting isolates of *E. coli*.

4. The spot indole test is a simple test which is used to presumptively identify *E. coli* isolates, especially from urine cultures. A positive spot indole test on an isolate which is beta-hemolytic and lactose fermenting is excellent evidence that the organism is *Escherichia coli*. Other organisms for which a positive spot indole test is frequently used to support a rapid identification are *Proteus vulgaris*, *Pasteurella multocida*, and *Propionibacterium acnes*.

5. The patient had a previous urinary tract infection, at which time she received oral ampicillin. One of the deleterious effects associated with the use of antimicrobial agents is the development of resistance. This occurs with some degree of frequency in the gut, where plasmids coding for resistance may be mobilized in response to antimicrobial pressure, leading to the transfer of resistance to previously susceptible organisms, such as in this *E. coli* isolate. Not only may resistance to the agent supplying the pressure result, but also the plasmid may contain genes which code for resistance to other antimicrobial agents, the end result being a multiple-drug-resistant organism. Since the gut has been shown to be an important reservoir for organisms causing urinary tract infection, resistance to ampicillin in the face of prior ampicillin therapy is not suprising.

6. The simplistic view of why women have more urinary tract infections than men is that the shorter urethra in women results in a greater likelihood that organisms will ascend the urethra and enter the bladder. However, other factors which may play a role in this gender difference have been identified. It has been observed that prostatic fluid inhibits the growth of common urinary tract pathogens in urine, providing a unique defense mechanism for men. It has also been observed that specific uropathogens bind to vaginal and periurethral epithelial cells. Binding in the periurethral region by these organisms is often seen in women prior to the development of urinary tract infection, as well as in women who have recurrent urinary tract infections. These observations may further explain why a preponderance of urinary tract infections are seen in women.

7. The clinical presentation in this patient is consistent with acute pyelonephritis. Pyelonephritis is an infection of the kidney, whereas cystitis is an infection of the bladder. The findings of fever, documented by a temperature of 38.8°C, chills, and left flank pain, with corresponding costovertebral angle tenderness, are all consistent with pyelonephritis. The patient's urinalysis and culture results would not be useful in differentiating be-

tween the two types of infections. Radiographic or cystoscopic studies would be necessary to make a definitive diagnosis of pyelonephritis, but clinical judgment is usually sufficient. The reason why it is important to distinguish between pyelonephritis and cystitis is that antimicrobial treatment strategies differ. Cystitis therapy is usually brief, often only a single dose of antimicrobial agents, whereas pyelonephritis therapy may be more prolonged, typically lasting 2 weeks.

REFERENCES

Johnson, J. R. 1991. Virulence factors in *Escherichia coli* urinary tract infections. *Clin. Microbiol. Rev.* **4**:80–128.

Stamm, W. E., G. W. Counts, K. R. Running, S. Fihn, M. Turck, and K. K. Holmes. 1982. Diagnosis of coliform infection in acutely dysuric women. *N. Engl. J. Med.* **307**:463–468.

Stark, R. P., and D. G. Maki. 1984. Bacteriuria in the catherized patient. What quantitative level of bacteriuria is relevant? *N. Engl. J. Med.* **311**:560–564.

The patient was a 19-year-old female. She was seen in the walk-in medicine clinic with complaints of right-knee and right-shoulder pain, nausea, and vomiting. On physical examination, she had a swollen right knee and decreased range of motion of her right shoulder. She also had a thick vaginal discharge. Her temperature was 38.4°C, and she had a WBC count of 15,700/mm^3. She gave a history of having two recent sexual partners. Blood, vaginal, and joint fluid cultures were performed. A Gram stain of joint fluid showed numerous polymorphonuclear cells, but no organisms were seen. Both the vaginal and joint fluid cultures were positive for the agent of infection.

1. What was the etiologic agent of her infection? What in her history supports this conclusion?

2. For which other agent(s) should the patient be examined? Explain your answer.

3. An empirical regimen of ceftriaxone was begun. What is an empirical antibiotic regimen? Why was ceftriaxone chosen to treat this infection?

4. This patient had a systemic infection. What phenotypic characteristics are found in isolates of this organism which cause systemic infections?

5. What should be done about her sexual partners?

DISCUSSION

1. This woman had septic arthritis due to *Neisseria gonorrhoeae*. The observations that the etiologic agent grew from vaginal discharge and that the patient had multiple sexual partners indicate that she was likely to have a sexually transmitted disease (STD).

   Arthritis is a fairly frequent complication of one of the STD agents, *N. gonorrhoeae*. It is estimated that between 0.5 and 3% of infected patients develop systemic infection and that the most common manifestation of systemic infection is septic arthritis.

2. Since this woman has an STD, she should be examined for *Chlamydia trachomatis* and *Treponema pallidum* (the agent of syphilis). Concurrent infections with these STD agents are frequent, and different therapies from those routinely used to treat *N. gonorrhoeae* are required to treat *C. trachomatis*. Because coinfection with gonococci and chlamydiae is so common, a combination of tetracycline (chlamydia therapy) and ceftriaxone (gonorrhea therapy) is routinely used therapeutically at STD clinics. Because this woman has engaged in high-risk behavior (unprotected intercourse with multiple sexual partners) for acquiring HIV infection, she should be screened for that agent as well. She should also be counseled regarding safe sexual practices.

3. The strategy of an empirical antibiotic regimen is to use an antimicrobial agent with a broad enough spectrum of activity to effectively treat the likely agents of a specific infection. In this case, ceftriaxone was chosen because of the high likelihood that this woman's infection was due to *N. gonorrhoeae*. Ceftriaxone has replaced penicillin G as the recommended treatment for all gonococcal infections. This is because an increasing number of *N. gonorrhoeae* isolates are becoming resistant to penicillin G. This resistance is due primarily to the ability of the organism to produce β-lactamase. β-Lactamase is a enzyme that breaks the beta-lactam ring of penicillin G, inactivating the antibiotic. In a survey of STD clinics throughout the United States, the number of β-lactamase-producing strains increased from 3.2 to 7.4% between 1988 and 1989. In the second half of 1990, approximately 25% of gonococcal isolates recovered at our institution were β-lactamase producers. Chromosomal mutation causing modification in penicillin-binding proteins has also led to penicillin G resistance. These strains are much more difficult to detect than the β-lactamase producers. This inability to reliably detect chromosomal resistance has further complicated the use of penicillin G to treat gonococcal infections.

4. Strains of *N. gonorrhoeae* that cause systemic infection usually are serum resistant; belong to the protein 1A serovar; usually are auxotrophic for

arginine, hypoxanthine, and uracil; and usually but not always are highly susceptible to penicillin G. A subpopulation of people who develop systemic infection with these strains have deficiencies in the terminal components of complement. People with this deficiency often have more than one episode of systemic gonococcal infection.

5. Both of her sexual partners should be notified to receive ceftriaxone treatment. If possible, their sexual partners should also be treated. These men should also be screened for other STDs outlined above in the discussion of question 2.

REFERENCES

Britigan, B. E., M. S. Cohen, and P. F. Sparling. 1985. Gonococcal infections: a model of molecular pathogenesis. *N. Engl. J. Med.* **312:**1683–1694.
Centers for Disease Control. 1990. Plasmid-mediated antimicrobial resistance in Neisseria gonorrhoeae—United States, 1988 and 1989. *Morbid. Mortal. Weekly Rep.* **39:**284–293.

CASE 20

This 23-year-old man presented to the emergency room with 3 days of pain-less urethral discharge. He had been sexually active with his girlfriend for the past 2 to 3 months. The patient noted a similar discharge 1 year prior to this visit, when he was having sexual relations with the same girlfriend. He denied fever, pain on urination, or inguinal adenopathy. Examination was remarkable for a white urethral discharge. Gram stain and culture for *Neisseria gonorrhoeae* were negative. A urethral culture was subsequently found to be positive for the causative agent.

1. What was the etiology of his infection? Which form of this organism is infectious? Why is this organism so frequently undiagnosed, especially in women?

2. What are some of the common complications associated with infections with this organism? Besides the genital tract, where else and in which population do infections with this organism occur?

3. How is the laboratory diagnosis of this organism made?

4. Why is ceftriaxone ineffective against this agent?

DISCUSSION

1. This patient had *Chlamydia trachomatis* urethritis. *C. trachomatis* is an obligate intracellular bacterium with a fairly complex life cycle. The organism has two forms, elementary bodies and reticulate bodies. The elementary body is the infectious, extracellular form of the organism, and the reticulate body is the intracellular, replicative form. Although the cell envelope of this organism is related to that of gram-negative organisms (having an inner and outer membrane), the organism is too small to observe by Gram stain.

   C. trachomatis is believed to be the most common agent of sexually transmitted disease (STD) in the United States, causing 3 to 4 million new cases each year. By comparison, it is estimated that there are approximately 700,000 to 800,000 new cases of gonorrhea (*N. gonorrhoeae*) and approximately 100,000 new cases of syphilis (*Treponema pallidum*) annually. *C. trachomatis* is underdiagnosed for at least three reasons. First, patients are often infected with more than one sexually transmitted disease (STD), obscuring the diagnosis of chlamydia. Unfortunately, therapies effective for gonorrhea and syphilis may not be effective for chlamydia (see the discussion of question 4), and if appropriate antichlamydial therapy is not used, the patient will remain infected. Second, *C. trachomatis* infection can frequently be mild or even asymptomatic, especially in women. The disease is usually self-limited. Many individuals may not realize they are infected unless they develop a symptomatic complication of their genital tract infection (see the discussion of question 2). Third, laboratory diagnosis of *C. trachomatis* infection can be difficult. Unlike *N. gonorrhoeae*, which can be frequently diagnosed in males by Gram stain, no diagnostic tool of comparable simplicity is available for *C. trachomatis*.

2. *C. trachomatis* can cause epididymitis. In individuals who practice receptive anal intercourse, it can cause proctitis and proctocolitis. The complications of genital tract infection in women tend to be more severe. Endometritis and salpingitis due to *C. trachomatis* may lead to pelvic inflammatory disease and sterility, especially in women who have had multiple chlamydial infections. Non-genital tract infections with this organism include pneumonia in infants and trachoma in adults. Infant pneumonia is probably obtained by vertical transmission. Conjunctivitis is seen in approximately one-half of infants with pneumonia. Trachoma is a chlamydial eye infection which causes keratoconjunctivitis. It is spread by direct contact with the eye, most probably via contaminated fingers. This infection is the leading cause of blindness worldwide, with infection occurring mainly in regions where poor personal hygiene is common.

3. A definitive diagnosis of *C. trachomatis* infection can be made in one of three ways: antibody-based techniques, culture, and DNA hybridization. (i) The organism can be detected directly in clinical specimens by using immunologically based techniques. Fluorescent monoclonal antibodies to elementary bodies are used to demonstrate *C. trachomatis* directly in clinical specimens. EIAs have been used as well. The two techniques are similar in sensitivity to culture. (ii) Because *C. trachomatis* is an obligate, intracellular parasite, tissue cell culture must be used to isolate this organism. *C. trachomatis* produces a characteristic cytoplasmic inclusion in these cells within 48 to 72 h, and fluorescent monoclonal antibodies can be used to confirm that the inclusion contains this organism. (iii) DNA hybridization with *C. trachomatis*-specific gene probes has been shown to be a rapid, sensitive, and specific means of detecting this organism.

4. Beta-lactam antimicrobial agents such as ceftriaxone have poor activity against *C. trachomatis* for two reasons. It is well known that beta-lactam antibotics are active only against growing bacteria and that they have poor intracellular penetration. The intracellular, replicative phase of *C. trachomatis* protects it from the activity of beta-lactam antibiotics. Second, although this organism has a cell envelope similar to gram-negative bacteria, investigators have been unable to demonstrate that it contains a peptidoglycan layer, the major cellular target for beta-lactam antibiotics. However, the organism does possess penicillin-binding protein, making it theoretically possible for beta-lactam antibiotics to kill it by means other than inhibition of peptidoglycan synthesis. Tetracyclines including doxycycline are the therapy of choice for this infection.

REFERENCES

Batteiger, B. E., and R. B. Jones. 1987. Chlamydial infections. *Infect. Dis. Clin. N. Am.* 1:55–82.
Hooton, T. M., and R. C. Barnes. 1987. Urethritis in men. *Infect. Dis. Clin. N. Am.* 1:165–178.
Stamm, W. E. 1988. Diagnosis of *Chlamydia trachomatis* genitourinary tract infections. *Ann. Intern. Med.* 108:710–717.

The patient is a 23-year-old male who works as a baker's assistant. He presented to the local emergency room with low-grade fever, malaise, and headache. He was sent home with a diagnosis of influenza. He presented 7 days later with a 1-day history of worsened headache, photophobia, and stiff neck. On physical examination he appeared to be in mild distress with a temperature of 38.8°C. He had mild nuchal rigidity and a maculopapular rash on his trunk, arms, palms, and soles. Areas on his palms and soles had some papulosquamous lesions. There were no mucous membrane lesions. No focal deficits were seen on neurologic examination. He had a white blood cell count of 11,200/mm^3 with an increased number of PMN. A computed tomogram (CT scan) of the head was normal, and a lumbar puncture revealed 120 white blood cells/mm^3 with 80% lymphocytes and 20% PMN, a glucose level of 40 mg/dl (normal), and a protein level of 82 mg/dl (elevated). Blood cultures were obtained, and antimicrobial therapy was begun. The next day a serologic test of his CSF and blood revealed the diagnosis. Further questioning of the patient when the serology results were known revealed that 1 month previously, he had a painless ulcer on his penis which healed spontaneously. His condition improved greatly over the next 3 days and his rash cleared within 10 days.

1. Which bacterial infections can cause a maculopapular rash?

2. What is the most likely agent of his infection?

3. In what stage of this infection is this patient? What is the significance of his CSF findings? Describe the disease course as it occurs in infected patients who go untreated.

4. How can the diagnosis of this infection be made? What is the difference between the screening test for the organism infecting this patient and the confirmatory test? How are these two tests used?

5. If this patient had been found to have a T-helper cell count of <200 and was HIV seropositive, what adjustment to his antimicrobial therapy would be necessary to treat the infection causing his skin rash?

DISCUSSION

1. A number of bacteria can cause a maculopapular rash. They include the
   rickettsias (the organisms that cause Rocky Mountain spotted fever and
   typhus), *Salmonella typhi, Borrelia burgdorferi* (the agent of Lyme disease),
   Neisseria gonorrhoeae, Leptospira spp., *Staphylococcus aureus* (the agent of
   toxic shock syndrome), the scarlet fever manifestation of group A streptococci, and *Treponema pallidum* (the agent of syphilis). In addition, a number
   of viral agents, including cytomegalovirus, measles virus, enteroviruses,
   parvovirus, and rubella virus, can cause maculopapular rashes. There are
   also numerous noninfectious causes of this particular type of rash. These
   rashes often represent an allergic reaction to specific drugs or foods.
   Alternatively, they may be seen in individuals with autoimmune disease
   (such as lupus) and sarcoid.

2. The history of having a painless penile ulcer, i.e., chancre, approximately 1
   month prior to the onset of his current symptoms is consistent with
   secondary syphilis. Because of his CNS findings, headache, photophobia,
   and stiff neck (nuchal rigidity), a lumbar puncture was performed. The
   findings of increased CSF protein and cell counts with a predominance of
   mononuclear cells are consistent with the aseptic meningitis manifestation of secondary syphilis. Patients with secondary syphilis infrequently
   (1 to 3%) have meningitis, but many (40%) can have CSF abnormalities
   without clinical disease of the CNS. His serologic results (see the discussion of question 4) were consistent with the diagnosis of syphilis.

3. The stages of syphilis are incubating, primary, secondary, latent, and late
   or tertiary. The incubating stage usually lasts for approximately 3 weeks
   after contact, usually sexual, with an infected individual. The primary
   stage is characterized by the development of the primary lesion, the
   chancre, at the site of infection. Many individuals, especially females, do
   not seek treatment because the lesions are painless and may not be visible
   if they are in the vagina or anal region. Untreated individuals progress to
   secondary syphilis. In this stage, a skin rash which begins on the trunk
   and spreads to the extremities including the palms and soles is seen in
   90% of patients. This manifestation is due to the dissemination of the
   spirochetes throughout the body. Skin lesions are teeming with spirochetes, so gloves should be worn when examining the skin rash in individuals with suspected secondary syphilis. Constitutional symptoms
   such as fever, malaise, and arthralgia are common. In this patient, the
   spirochetes invaded the central nervous system as well.

   After resolution of the secondary stage of the disease, the infection
   enters the latent phase. These individuals are asymptomatic but still have

evidence of disease based on the presence of specific antibodies to *T. pallidum.*

Latent syphilis develops into late or tertiary syphilis in approximately 30% of untreated individuals. This stage of the disease occurs years after resolution of the secondary stage. The most severe manifestations of late syphilis are neurosyphilis and cardiovascular syphilis. Two of the most important findings in neurosyphilis are general paresis and tabes dorsalis. Late syphilis, especially of the cardiovascular system, is encountered infrequently now that penicillin has been established as a safe and effective therapy for syphilis.

4. Syphilis can be diagnosed in two different ways. The spirochete can be directly detected in lesions of patients with primary and secondary syphilis. This is done by dark-field microscopy examination of tissue scrapings for the presence of treponemes. This technique requires a dark-field microscope and individuals skilled in its use. It is usually performed only in settings such as sexually transmitted disease clinics, where large numbers of potientally infected individuals are available for study.

The diagnosis is usually made serologically. Initially a VDRL (Venereal Disease Research Laboratory) or RPR (rapid plasma reagin) screening test is performed. These two tests detect antibodies to reagin, which is an antigen present in patients with syphilis. This antigen is believed to be produced as a result of the interaction of *T. pallidum* with the patient's tissue. The characteristics of a good screening test are rapidity, ease of performance, and low cost. These characteristics are important because they permit large populations to be tested cheaply and efficiently. The screening test should also be highly sensitive (all the patients with the disease are detected), but they do not have to be highly specific (not all patients with a positive test have the disease). Both the VDRL and RPR tests meet the criteria of a good screening test, although it should be understood that a positive VDRL or RPR test does not necessarily confirm *T. pallidum* infection. The reason is that patients with other disease states, both infectious and autoimmune, can have a positive VDRL or RPR test. In the primary stage of the disease the test is 70 to 80% sensitive; in secondary disease, the sensitivity approaches 100%. Patients who have positive results in one of these two serologic tests should have a confirmatory test done. The most important characteristic of a confirmatory test is that it be highly specific; i.e., those with a positive confirmatory test truly have the disease. Confirmatory tests are more complicated, time-consuming, and expensive than screening tests. The confirmatory tests used for syphilis diagnosis are FTA-abs (fluorescent treponeme antibody-absorbed), MHA-TP (microhemagglutination assay-*T. pallidum*), and TPHA (*T. pal-*

lidum hemagglutination assay). All are dependent on detecting antibodies which bind specifically to *T. pallidum,* and, as such, all are highly specific. All patients with secondary syphilis have a positive serum FTA-abs, TPHA, or MHA-TP test, and these antibodies will be detectable throughout the patient's life.

5. If this patient had had a T-helper cell count of $<200/mm^3$ and a serologic test positive for HIV, he would be defined as having AIDS. Syphilis is much more difficult to eradicate in patients with AIDS because of their defect in cell-mediated immunity. If prolonged antimicrobial therapy is not used in these patients, treatment may fail. AIDS patients with syphilis must be carefully monitored after the completion of therapy so that relapses or treatment failures can be identified.

REFERENCES

Hook, E. W., III. 1989. Syphilis and HIV infection. *J. Infect. Dis.* **160:**530–534.
Musher, D. M. 1987. Syphilis. *Infect. Dis. Clin. N. Am.* **1:**83–95.

The patient was a 3-year-old male. On the day of admission, he complained of a headache and developed fever with lethargy and emesis. He had a 2-day history of a mild upper respiratory illness. On admission, he had a fever of 39.7°C and was extremely lethargic, responsive only to deep pain. A lumbar puncture revealed 21,000 WBC/mm^3 with 90% polymorphonuclear cells, a CSF glucose level of 9 mg/dl (normal, 40 to 80 mg/dl), and a CSF protein level of 1,322 mg/dl (normal, 15 to 45 mg/dl). The Gram stain of CSF was positive for numerous white cells and gram-negative coccobacilli. (See Figure 7.) A CSF antigen detection test was positive for the same organism.

1. What was the clinical diagnosis in this patient? Which organisms commonly cause this type of infection in this age group? What organism is causing his infection?

2. Which organisms are detected in a CSF antigen detection test? Which antigen is generally detected? In which clinical situations do these tests have their greatest value?

3. Why are children 2 months to 5 years of age susceptible to infection with this organism?

4. How can this infection be prevented?

5. How might the child's upper respiratory tract infection have contributed to his development of systemic illness?

DISCUSSION

1. This patient has bacterial meningitis. The finding of an extremely high white blood cell count (normal, 0 to 3 cells) and CSF protein level in conjunction with a low CSF glucose level and a positive Gram stain is indicative of this type of infection. All the CSF parameters are inconsistent with both viral and fungal meningitis. The most common etiologic agent of bacterial meningitis in a 3-year-old child is *Haemophilus influenzae* type b. The Gram stain of CSF is consistent with meningitis due to this organism and culture of his CSF was positive for it. Other important agents of bacterial meningitis in children 2 months to 5 years of age are *Streptococcus pneumoniae* (gram-positive cocci) and *Neisseria meningitidis* (gram-negative diplococci).

2. Antigen detection tests have been developed for the most common agents of bacterial meningitis, including *H. influenzae* type b, group B streptococci, *S. pneumoniae*, and *N. meningitidis*. Generally speaking, the capsular polysaccharide is detected in this test. Latex particle agglutination is widely used for bacterial antigen detection. In this test, latex particles are sensitized (coated) with antisera specific for one of these bacterial antigens. The sensitized particles are mixed with CSF, serum, or urine, and the presence of agglutination indicates the presence of a specific antigen. In this case, latex particles sensitized with antibodies against polyribosylphosphate (PRP), the capsular polysaccharide of *H. influenzae* type b, reacted with this antigen present in CSF. This antigen is also excreted in urine and could have been found in that body fluid as well. Antigen is also present in serum. Serum is infrequently used in antigen detection for agents of bacterial meningitis because it can cause nonspecific agglutination. In this particular case, given the child's age and Gram-stain findings, *H. influenzae* is the most likely agent; therefore antigen detection is of little value in this clinical situation and should not have been done. Bacterial antigen detection is most useful in two clinical situations. One situation occurs when the patient is treated with antimicrobial agents before a CSF specimen is obtained. In this setting, culture and CSF Gram stain may be negative but antigen detection tests may be positive, helping to guide the choice of antimicrobial therapy. The second situation is in children between 2 weeks and 3 months of age who have a CSF Gram stain positive for gram-positive diplococci. Since two agents, group B streptococci and *S. pneumoniae*, may be likely causes of the meningitis, antigen detection can be useful in rapidly distinguishing between them.

3. To optimally ward off infection with encapsulated bacteria such as *H. influenzae* type b, individuals must mount a humoral (antibody) response

against the capsular material, which is generally but not always a polysaccharide. The major pathogenic activity of the *H. influenzae* type b capsule is to prevent phagocytosis of the organism. When antibodies bind to the capsule, they reverse its antiphagocytic activity such that white blood cells are stimulated to phagocytize and kill these bacteria.

Children less than 2 months of age maintain a humoral response to these encapsulated organisms by virtue of having received these antibodies transplacentally. Between 2 months and 2 years of age, children are often not able to mount a protective humoral response to polysaccharide antigens such as capsules and are therefore prone to infections with encapsulated agents. Investigators have shown that the serum of children between 3 months and 3 years does not have bactericidal activity against *H. influenzae* type b, making them susceptible to infection with this organism. The large majority of systemic *H. influenzae* infections occur in children in this age group. Children between 3 and 5 years of age who get serious infections with this organism may not yet have mounted a protective antibody response, although almost all children are immune by their fourth birthday.

4. A protective vaccine has recently been developed. It consists of PRP derived from the capsule of *H. influenzae* type b coupled with either diphtheria or tetanus toxoid. This combination vaccine is now approved for use in infants with the initial series of vaccinations at 2, 4, and 6 months of age and with booster doses at 15 months of age and before entering school. Infants and young children (<18 months) are frequently unable to mount an adequate immune response against T-cell-independent antigens such as capsular polysaccharide. When the polysaccharide antigen is conjugated with diphtheria or tetanus toxoid, the conjugate becomes a T-cell-dependent antigen owing to the presence of the protein toxoid. Infants and young children have been shown to be quite capable of mounting protective immune responses to T-cell-dependent antigens. Recent preliminary studies suggest that institution of *H. influenzae* type b vaccine programs has significantly reduced the number of cases of meningitis.

5. The respiratory tract is often the initial site of infection in patients who develop systemic disease with *H. influenzae* type b. In a small percentage of children, the organism enters the bloodstream from the respiratory tract and causes bacteremia. It must be emphasized that organisms causing systemic infection are almost always encapsulated and that *H. influenzae* encapsulated with type b polysaccharide accounts for over 90% of the cases of *H. influenzae* bacteremia. In a smaller percentage still, the organism may invade the meninges and cause meningitis. Other systemic infec-

tions with this organism include buccal cellulitis, septic arthritis, and epiglottitis.

REFERENCES

Anderson, P., R. Johnston, and D. H. Smith. 1972. Human sera activities against *H. influenzae* type b. *J. Clin. Invest.* **51**:31–38.

Hoban, J., E. Witnicki, and G. W. Hammonds. 1985. Bacterial antigen detection in cerebrospinal fluid of patients with meningitis. *Diagn. Microbiol. Infect. Dis.* **3**:373–379.

A 3½-year-old male presented to an outside emergency room with fever and lethargy since the previous evening and a petechial rash first noted on the day of evaluation. On physical examination the patient was listless and had a temperature of 39°C, blood pressure of 104/52 mmHg, and heart rate of 148 beats/min. Examination of the skin revealed a petechial rash as well as two purpuric lesions. Blood cultures were obtained, and he was given intravenous antibiotics and transferred to this hospital. On arrival here, he underwent a lumbar puncture, which was notable for cerebrospinal fluid with 190 white blood cells/mm^3, with 94% neutrophils, consistent with bacterial meningitis. No organisms were seen on Gram stain of the cerebrospinal fluid. Blood cultures from the outside hospital were subsequently positive for an oxidase-positive, gram-negative diplococcus.

1. Which bacterium was causing this patient's illness? Is the finding of meningitis a positive or negative prognostic sign in this patient? Explain your answer.

2. Is this organism ever part of the normal oropharyngeal flora? Explain your answer.

3. Which immunologic abnormalities predispose individuals to infection with this organism?

4. Which serogroup(s) causes illness? The serogroup is based on antigen from which part of the bacterium?

5. Which prophylactic strategies are useful for large populations?

6. Which prophylactic strategies can be used for exposed individuals?

7. What are purpuric lesions and a petechial rash, and which virulence factor plays a central role responsible for their appearance?

DISCUSSION

1. The clinical presentation, the finding of meningitis (190 white blood cells/ mm^3, primarily neutrophils, in the CSF), and the finding of oxidase-positive, gram-negative diplococci growing in the blood strongly indicated that the etiologic agent of this infection was *Neisseria meningitidis*. This organism is a frequent cause of meningitis in this patient population. Recent data from the Centers for Disease Control (CDC) indicate that *Haemophilus influenzae* is the most frequent cause of meningitis in this age group, whereas *N. meningitidis* and *Streptococcus pneumoniae* cause significantly fewer cases.

   The finding of meningitis in this patient, although grave, is actually an encouraging prognostic sign. The reason for this is that fulminant disease can occur with this organism. In these cases, the disease course from initial symptoms to death can be measured in hours. Patients with fulminant disease often will die before developing signs and symptoms of meningitis. The findings of meningitis, then, indicates that the course of disease has not been so rapid to preclude its development. The most recently reported case fatality rate for *N. meningitidis* meningitis from the CDC is 13%. It is higher for fulminant meningococcemia.

2. *N. meningitidis* is usually considered to be part of the oropharyngeal flora and can be found in 20 to 40% of healthy young adults. During epidemics of meningococcal disease in institutionalized populations such as the military, colonization rates may approach 90%.

3. Most people who are colonized with this organism mount a humoral response to it. These individuals produce bactericidal antibodies, which appear to be protective. The very small percentage of patients who do not make bactericidal antibodies in response to colonization by this organism are at high risk for development of invasive disease. Some patients who make antibodies have deficiencies in the terminal components of the complement pathway, and therefore these antibodies may not be bactericidal, nor can the alternative complement pathway be triggered. This complement deficiency places them at risk for disseminated disease as well. Finally, asplenic individuals are thought to be at increased risk for infection with this organism.

4. The serogroups most commonly associated with meningitis in the United States are types A, C, Y, W135, and B. The two most frequently isolated serogroups are B (50%) and C (20%). Typically groups A and C are thought of as epidemic strains because of their association with epidemics, whereas group B isolates are more likely to cause sporadic cases. Cases due to group B are most frequent because of the rarity of epidemics of *N. menin-*

gitidis disease in the United States. The serogroups are based on the biochemical structure of the capsular polysaccharide that surrounds the organism. Nonencapsulated isolates rarely cause invasive disease, indicating that encapsulation is critical to the pathogenicity of the organism.

5. Vaccination is the mainstay of prophylactic strategies for large populations. Vaccines derived from capsular polysaccharide are highly protective against groups A and C in adults and children over 2 years of age. The duration of immunity does not exceed 3 years; it is longer for group A than group C. A quadrivalent vaccine for groups A, C, Y, and W135 has been developed. Its efficacy is not yet known, although antibody responses are better for groups A and C than groups Y and W135. No vaccine is currently available for group B meningococci because of the poor immunogenicity of their capsular polysaccharide.

6. Both vaccination and chemoprophylaxis may be in order for exposed individuals, especially health care workers who come in close contact with respiratory secretions of infected individuals. Rifampin is the drug of choice for antimicrobial prophylaxis. It penetrates well into respiratory secretions and is well tolerated. The purpose of chemoprophylaxis is twofold. One is to protect the individual receiving the drug. The second is to eliminate nasopharyngeal carriage of the organism to limit its spread in the general population. However, cases of meningococcal meningitis in patients given rifampin prophylaxis have been reported. These isolates were found to be rifampin resistant. In addition, rifampin will not eliminate carriage in 10 to 20% of colonized individuals.

   Two practical points concern rifampin prophylaxis. First, patients should be informed that it causes secretions to turn orange. Urine, breast milk, and tears will all be affected, and contact lenses can be permanently stained by this drug. Second, pharmacies in rural areas may not stock this drug, making it inconvenient to get and thus adversely affecting compliance. Arrangements should be made to ensure that contacts can obtain this drug.

7. Petechial rash and purpuric lesions can be manifestations of disseminated intravascular coagulation (DIC). Petechial lesions are pinpoint, purplish red lesions that are caused by hemorrhage in the intradermal vascular bed. Purpuric lesions are similar to petechial lesions but are larger, probably representing coalescence of a number of petechial lesions. Endotoxin found in the outer membrane of *N. meningitidis* is a well-recognized mediator of DIC.

REFERENCES

Peltola, H. 1983. Meningococcal disease: still with us. *Rev. Infect. Dis.* **5:**71–91.
Schlech, W. F., III, J. I. Ward, J. D. Band, A. Hightower, D. W. Fraser, and C. V. Broome. 1985. Bacterial meningitis in the United States, 1978 to 1981. The national bacterial meningitis surveillance study. *JAMA* **253:**1749–1754.

The patient was a 2,150-g female neonate born at 32 weeks gestation. Her Apgar scores were 2 and 7, and she was intubated at birth because of poor respiratory effort. The mother presented at the time of delivery with complaints of lower abdominal pain with a temperature of 39°C and white blood cell count of 25,000/mm^3. The mother was given ampicillin at the time of delivery. Blood cultures taken from the infant soon after birth grew grampositive coccobacilli. Two lumbar punctures were attempted, which were traumatic.

1. On the basis of the Gram stain and the patient's age, which two organisms are likely? Which simple biochemical test can be used to differentiate isolated colonies of these two organisms?

2. Which data in the case report indicate that the mother had an infection? What is the likely outcome of this infection for the mother?

3. What is the epidemiology of the organism in pregnant women? in neonates? Which other populations can be infected with this organism?

4. How is a traumatic lumbar puncture detected? Because of the traumatic lumbar puncture, a positive cerebrospinal fluid culture would not necessarily be indicative of meningitis in this patient. Explain this statement.

DISCUSSION

1. This child has *Listeria monocytogenes* bacteremia. The two most common agents of neonatal bacteremia are this organism and group B streptococci. Group B streptococci are gram-positive diplococci which on Gram stain can be confused with *L. monocytogenes*. Further complicating matters is the fact that on sheep blood agar these two organisms have similar colony morphologies and both produce a narrow zone of beta-hemolysis around individual colonies. They can easily be distinguished by the catalase test. *L. monocytogenes* is catalase positive whereas group B streptococci are catalase negative.

2. The mother's high fever and white blood cell count are both indicative of infection. Ampicillin was given to the mother because both *L. monocytogenes* and group B streptococci are susceptible to this agent and are common causes of bacteremia in pregnancy. Not only is the mother's infection treated, but also this therapy is used as prophylaxis for the infant. These infections are generally self-limited in the mothers but can have devastating consequences for the child.

3. *L. monocytogenes* can be a member of the normal bowel flora, and for reasons that are not entirely clear it can pass through the bowel wall and cause bacteremia in both pregnant women and immunocompromised patients. Outbreaks of systemic infection following ingestion of contaminated foods are well documented in these two populations as well. Dairy products seem to be an important vehicle for this organism, with two disease outbreaks being traced to soft cheese and ice cream bars. One of the important characteristics of this organism which may explain its predilection for these foods is its ability to replicate at refrigeration temperatures (2 to 8°C). Vertical transmission from mother to child is an extremely important mode of spread of this organism. The organism can be transmitted transplacentally, leading to stillbirth, septic abortion, or premature delivery of the fetus. The organism can also be transmitted at birth while the baby is passing through a colonized birth canal. Children who are infected in utero or during passage through the birth canal often are ill at birth or become symptomatic within 3 days of birth. These children are classified as having early-onset disease. In premature infants, this disease is associated with a very high mortality. The main focus of the infection is the lungs in children with bacteremia. With *L. monocytogenes* obtained in utero, multiple abscesses can also be seen in any organ of the reticuloendothelial system including the liver or spleen, as well as the kidneys and even the brain. Late-onset disease due to *L. monocytogenes* or group B streptococci generally occurs 10 to 14 days after birth but may occur up to

2 months after birth. The actual source of infection is unknown and may represent nosocomial acquisition of these organisms. A major focus of infection is the central nervous system, with meningoencephalitis being frequent. The mortality is not as high as for early-onset disease, but is still significant.

4. A traumatic lumbar puncture usually contains gross blood, and the ratio of red blood cells (RBCs) to white blood cells in the CSF is similar to that seen in blood, approximately 500 to 1,000 RBCs to 1 WBC. A positive culture of CSF in this setting may actually represent bacteremia with the blood "contaminating" the CSF. If bacteremic blood is inoculated into the CSF by the lumbar puncture, the end result can be meningitis.

REFERENCES

Ciesielski, C. A., A. W. Hightower, S. K. Parsons, and C. V. Broome. 1988. Listeriosis in the United States: 1980-1982. *Arch. Intern. Med.* **148:**1416–1419.

Marget, W., and H. P. R. Seeliger. 1988. *Listeria monocytogenes* infections: therapeutic possibilities and problems. *Infection* **16:**S175–S177.

Schwartz, B., D. Hexter, C. V. Broome, A. W. Hightower, R. B. Hirschhorn, J. D. Porter, P. S. Hayes, W. F. Bibb, B. Lorber, and D. G. Faris. 1989. Investigation of an outbreak of listeriosis: new hypotheses for the etiology of epidemic *Listeria monocytogenes* infections. *J. Infect. Dis.* **159:**680–685.

This 65-year-old woman was bitten by her cat on the dorsal aspect of the right middle finger at 8:00 a.m. She rinsed the bite with water, and at 4:30 p.m. she noted pain and swelling in the finger and the dorsum of the right hand. She then noted pain in the axilla, red streaking up the forearm, and chills. On examination, she had a temperature of 38°C and her right upper extremity was notable for swelling, erythema, warmth, and tenderness on the dorsum of the hand. Two small puncture wounds were seen on the proximal phalanx of the long finger, and erythema was visible over the extensor surface of the forearm. Axillary tenderness was also noted. Laboratory studies demonstrated an elevated white blood cell count of 12,000/mm^3 with a left shift (the presence of immature neutrophils in peripheral blood). Aspiration of an abscess on her finger was sent for culture, and the patient was taken to the operating room for incision and drainage of the abscess. An oxidase-positive gram-negative coccobacillus that grew on chocolate agar but not on MacConkey agar was recovered from the abscess.

1. Which organism was isolated on culture of the abscess?

2. What is the reservoir of this organism? How do humans most commonly become infected by this organism?

3. How can infection with this organism be prevented?

4. Which other clinical syndromes can be caused by this organism?

DISCUSSION

1. The organism that was isolated from this patient's abscess was *Pasteurella multocida*. Another gram-negative coccobacillus that grows on chocolate agar but not on MacConkey agar and is frequently encountered clinically is *Haemophilus influenzae*. This organism, however, is unlikely to be associated with a wound infection and abscess following an animal bite. Another feature of this case which is typical for *P. multocida* is the rapid onset of infection following animal bites.

2. *P. multocida* is widely distributed throughout nature and is part of the normal flora in the nasopharynx of many mammals (both wild and domestic) and birds. Human infection is most likely to be associated with cat bites or scratches and less likely to be caused by dog bites. Infections following bites by other members of the cat family, including lions, have been reported to cause *P. multocida* wound infections and are occupational hazards for zoo keepers and veterinarians. In a minority of human infections the patients have had no known animal exposure.

3. Infection can be prevented by limiting contact with cats and dogs. If a person is bitten, the wound should be thoroughly cleaned as soon as is possible.

4. In addition to soft tissue infection with rapid onset, other infections seen with this organism following animal bite include osteomyelitis, tenosynovitis, abscess formation, and arthritis. Serious infections are more frequent following cat rather than dog bites. It is speculated that the cat tooth, which is long and thin, causes wounds that more readily puncture the tendon sheath (tenosynovitis) or periosteum (osteomyelitis). These infections are particularly problematic because they often occur on the hands and wrists. Because of the extraordinarily complex anatomy involved, infections of the hand and wrist, if neglected, can require complicated surgical debridement and loss of important motor function for the patient either temporarily or permanently. Other unusual complications include bacteremia with septic shock, meningitis, brain abscess, and peritonitis.

REFERENCES

Weber, D. J., and A. R. Hansen. 1991. Infections resulting from animal bites. *Infect. Dis. Clin. N. Am.* 5:663–680.
Weber, D. J., J. S. Wolfson, and M. N. Swartz. 1984. *Pasteurella multocida* infections: report of 34 cases and a review of the literature. *Medicine* 63:133–154.

This 53-year-old slaughterhouse worker was in excellent health until 8 weeks prior to admission, when he developed a flulike syndrome with fever, cough, nausea, vomiting, and anorexia. Although his symptoms abated, he noted a 40-lb (18-kg) weight loss over the following 8 weeks. Two weeks prior to admission, he noted early morning shaking chills with fevers and night sweats. He was referred for evaluation of fever and weight loss.

On examination he was febrile to 39.8°C and was having a shaking chill. The physical examination was otherwise unremarkable. Laboratory studies were notable for anemia (hematocrit of 34%). PPD and intradermal skin tests for blastomycin, histoplasmin, and coccidioidin were negative. A liver biopsy specimen contained granulomas. Blood cultures taken on the first two hospital days were subsequently found to be positive after prolonged incubation.

1. This patient had a fever of unknown origin (FUO). List five organisms commonly included in the differential diagnosis of this syndrome.

2. How would knowing his occupation help you narrow the list of possible agents?

3. The organism recovered from blood was a gram-negative, pleomorphic coccobacillus that was rapidly urease positive (20 min), oxidase positive, and unable to ferment glucose. Of the organisms you listed in your answer to question 2, which one is this?

4. Why are bone marrow cultures helpful in diagnosis of the etiologic agent in people with FUOs?

DISCUSSION

1. An FUO is exactly as it sounds. The patient has a fever which cannot be explained. Generally speaking, the patient is hospitalized with fevers for at least 1 week before being classified as having an FUO. Approximately 30 to 40% of FUOs in adults (slightly more in children) are due to infection. Neoplasms, especially lymphoma and leukemia, are important causes of FUO. Other noninfectious etiologies responsible for prolonged and unexplained fevers are inflammatory bowel disease, autoimmune disease such as lupus erythematosus and rheumatoid arthritis, and sarcoid.

   The source of infection in FUO is, as a rule, extremely difficult to identify. Abscesses, osteomyelitis, bacterial endocarditis, and biliary and urinary tract infections are all potential sources of FUO. These sites are often infected with organisms that represent the contiguous normal flora (gut flora in abdominal or liver abscess, etc.). Occasionally FUOs are due to organisms which are more difficult to grow and/or are infrequently encountered as etiologies of infection; some of these represent the endogenous flora, and others are obtained exogenously. Some of these organisms which can be a challenge for the clinical laboratory to detect and are considered in the differential diagnosis of FUO include *Mycobacterium tuberculosis* and *M. avium* complex (the latter is usually a cause of FUO only in AIDS patients), *Salmonella typhi*, *Francisella tularensis*, *Borrelia* spp. (including the Lyme disease agent, *B. burgdorferi*), *Rickettsia* spp., *Coxiella burnetii* (the agent of Q fever), *Chlamydia psittaci*, *Leptospira* spp., the HACEK organisms (*Haemophilus aphrophilus*, *Actinobacillus actinomycetemcomitans*, *Cardiobacterium hominis*, *Eikenella corrodens*, and *Kingella kingii*), *Treponema pallidum* (the agent of syphilis), and *Brucella* spp. Other infectious agents including fungi, viruses, and parasites must also be taken into consideration. Many of the agents on this list cause "culture-negative" endocarditis, and FUOs may be a manifestation of this disease.

   This patient's clinical course (night sweats, fever, large weight loss) is most consistent with tuberculosis. However, his negative PPD test and no mention of an abnormal chest radiograph make this diagnosis less likely but still possible.

2. Being a slaughterhouse worker means that he will have a much greater likelihood of exposure to organisms which cause zoonotic infections. In particular, he would be at increased risk for infection with *Brucella* spp. Other organisms that cause FUOs for which he may have higher exposure rates than the general population include *Salmonella* spp., *Mycobacterium* spp., *Campylobacter* spp., *Listeria monocytogenes*, and *Coxiella burnetii*. If he worked in a poultry-processing plant, *Chlamydia psittaci* and fungi such as

Histoplasma capsulatum (from poultry manure and crates) should also be added to the above list.

3. On the basis of the characteristics of this organism, it is most likely to be *Brucella* spp. The extremely rapid urease reaction is typical of *Brucella suis*. Although not stated in the case, the assumption is that he probably slaughtered pigs since *B. suis* infection is most frequently associated with exposure to infected pigs.

4. Several organisms that are in the differential diagnosis of FUO can produce foci of infection in the bone marrow. These organisms typically cause granulomas not only in bone marrow but also in other organs of the reticuloendothelial system such the liver (as was seen in this patient), spleen, lungs, or lymph nodes. Most of these agents are facultative or obligate intracellular parasites, including *Brucella* spp., *Salmonella* spp., and *Mycobacterium* spp. For example, in patients with typhoid fever, bone marrow cultures have a higher positive yield than do cultures of peripheral blood. Therefore, cultures of bone marrow in addition to cultures of blood may increase the likelihood of detecting the etiologic agent of FUOs.

REFERENCES

Dinarello, C. A., and S. M. Wolff. 1990. Fever of unknown origin, p. 468–478. *In* G. L. Mandell, R. G. Douglas, Jr., and J. E. Bennett (ed.), *Principles and Practice of Infectious Diseases,* 3rd ed. Churchill Livingstone, Inc., New York.
Petersdorf, R. G., and P. B. Beeson. 1961. Fever of unexplained origin. *Medicine* **40:**1–30.

This 40-year-old female noted an ulcer on the distal aspect of her right third finger approximately 12 days prior to admission. She developed chills and fever and was treated with oral antibiotics without success; she was then referred for admission to this hospital. On physical examination, the patient was an obese female in moderate distress. Her temperature was 40°C, her blood pressure was 146/82 mmHg, her pulse was 120 beats/min, and her respiration was 18/min. Remarkable physical findings included an excoriated, ulcerated lesion of the right third finger and associated epitrochlear and axillary adenopathy (enlarged lymph nodes). Cultures (including blood and wound surface) were negative. Retrospective questioning revealed that the patient had butchered a rabbit 1 week prior to the onset of her illness.

1. Which pathogen is the most likely agent of infection on the basis of the rabbit exposure?

2. Give two reasons why the laboratory must be notified in advance when attempting to isolate this organism from tissue.

3. Serologic means of making the diagnosis were attempted in this patient. Her initial titer against this bacterium was 320, and a follow-up titer 2 weeks later was 2,560. How much of a rise in titer does this represent, and does such a rise in titer indicate disease?

4. Describe four different clinical manifestations of infection with this organism. How is each manifestation of the disease contracted?

DISCUSSION

1. This infection is an example of a zoonotic infection. The organism most likely to cause rabbit-associated infections is *Francisella tularensis*, the etiologic agent of tularemia. Tularemia has also been referred to as "rabbit skinner disease" or "rabbit fever" because of its strong association with this animal. Infection with this organism is also transmitted by ticks. More than 100 species of animals are known to be infected by this organism. The organism is a very small, fastidious, gram-negative coccobacillus. Infection with *F. tularensis* was confirmed by serology in this case (see the answer to question 3).

2. The laboratory must be notified for two reasons. First and foremost, this organism is easily aerosolized and is highly infectious. Therefore specimens suspected of containing *F. tularensis* must be handled in some type of biological safety cabinet. Culture plates should be sealed and examined only in a safety cabinet. Secondary infections of laboratory workers have been reported. Second, this organism has special growth requirements. Blood agar enriched with cystine and chocolate agar enriched with IsoVitaleX (a commercially available mixture of vitamins and other microbial growth factors) both support the growth of this organism, and their use is necessary to ensure recovery of the organism. However, the organism can be difficult to recover from clinical specimens, and, as was seen in this case, alternative methods (serology) may be required to make the diagnosis of tularemia.

3. This woman had an eightfold rise in her titer against *F. tularensis*. A fourfold rise in titer over a 2-week period would be consistent with an acute infection with this organism. In fact, an individual with a single titer of 1:160 or higher, as was seen with her initial serologic examination, would be considered to be infected. A rising titer over time is more convincing as a diagnostic test than is a single titer because *F. tularensis* cross-reacts with a variety of microorganisms and a single, high titer may represent a cross-reaction. Concurrent *Brucella* titers (the organism with which *F. tularensis* is most likely to cross-react) may aid in interpretation of these serologic tests.

4. There are several different clinical manifestations of infection with *F. tularensis*. This patient had the ulceroglandular form of the disease with an ulcerated skin lesion and enlarged regional lymph nodes. She obtained this infection via direct contact with an infected rabbit. The most frequent manner in which ulceroglandular disease, the most common manifestation of tularemia, is obtained is via the bite of an infected tick, mosquito, or deerfly (vector-borne disease). In vector-borne disease, the ulcers are

usually located on the lower extremities, trunk, or head rather than the hand. The glandular form of the disease is usually vector borne. In this form of the disease, there may be enlarged lymph nodes as well as constitutional symptoms (fever, malaise), but no skin lesions. Another form of tularemia is oculoglandular disease. Patients directly inoculate the conjunctiva either by rubbing the eye with an infected hand or by aerosolization from infected material such as animal carcasses. They develop a painful, purulent conjunctivitis with cervical and preauricular lymphadenopathy.

Typhoidal tularemia is the most severe manifestation of the disease. This occurs following ingestion of contaminated water or undercooked, infected meat; by aerosol exposure; or by direct contact. The patients have fever, weight loss, and pneumonia with a nonproductive cough but no lymphadenopathy. This disease can mimic typhoid fever, brucellosis, and tuberculosis. It also has significant mortality (5 to 10%).

REFERENCES

Craven, R. B., and A. M. Barnes. 1991. Plague and tularemia. *Infect. Dis. Clin. N. Am.* 5:165–175.

Weinberg, A. N. 1991. Respiratory infections transmitted from animals. *Infect. Dis. Clin. N. Am.* 5:649–661.

CASE **28**

This 21-year-old man presented to the emergency room with 3 days of abdominal pain, which began as a diffuse, dull, continuous pain. The pain became crampy in the midgastric and lower abdomen. He noted a decrease in appetite but no nausea, vomiting, or diarrhea. On examination, the patient was febrile to 39.2°C, tachycardic with a heart rate of 150 beats/min, and tachypneic with a respiratory rate of 52/min and had a blood pressure of 108/60 mmHg. His physical examination was notable for midgastric and right lower quadrant abdominal tenderness. The white blood cell count was normal. Blood cultures were obtained on admission and were subsequently positive for an anaerobic, gram-negative rod, at which time the patient was taken to the operating room for an exploratory laparotomy.

1. To which genus do you think this organism belongs and why?

2. Upon learning of the positive blood culture, the surgical team opted for abdominal surgery. What type of lesion would you suspect they would find in the abdomen?

3. How is this intra-abdominal lesion treated?

4. What would surgical samples of this lesion be likely to grow on culture?

5. What other types of infections does this organism cause?

DISCUSSION

1. Anaerobic, nonsporeforming, gram-negative rods include the *Bacteroides* species and the *Fusobacterium* species. This patient had bacteremia with *Bacteroides fragilis*. There are a number of clinically important *Bacteroides* species, with *Bacteroides fragilis* being the most important. This organism is part of the normal colonic flora of humans.

2. *B. fragilis* is often involved in forming intra-abdominal (and intrapelvic) abscesses. Given that the patient had a positive blood culture for this organism, a likely explanation for the positive blood culture was thought to be an intra-abdominal abscess. At laparotomy, this patient was found to have a gangrenous appendix and 1,000 ml of purulent fluid within his abdomen. Whenever a patient has bacteremia, it is crucial to determine its source.

    B. fragilis is commonly involved in the formation of an abscess following perforation of the intestine. Animal studies have shown that abscess formation occurs most frequently when both anaerobic and facultative gram-negative rods are introduced into the intra-abdominal space. The combination of *B. fragilis* and *Escherichia coli*, in particular, is very efficient in inducing abscess formation.

3. Treatment of an intra-abdominal abscess involves a combination of drainage of the abscess (which may be performed either by surgery or percutaneously with radiologic guidance) and the administration of antibiotics. Antibiotic therapy alone is not reliable since there is no blood flow at the center of an abscess to deliver the antibiotics and the low pH and anaerobic conditions present in an abscess inactivate certain antibiotics.

4. Given the pathogenesis of intra-abdominal abscess described in the answer to question 2, most abscesses are polymicrobial. Since colonic contents contain numerous anaerobic and aerobic bacteria, it should come as no surprise that cultures from an abscess often reflect the normal colonic flora. Both *B. fragilis* and *E. coli*, as well as *Fusobacterium* species, were recovered from cultures of the intra-abdominal abscess of this patient. All these organisms are part of the normal colonic flora, and all three can grow under anaerobic conditions.

5. In addition to intra-abdominal abscesses (including liver abscesses, subphrenic abscesses, etc.), *B. fragilis* can be cultured from pelvic abscesses (including tuboovarian abscesses). It should be recognized that pelvic abscess can be a complication of gynecologic surgery and that intra-abdominal abscess can follow abdominal surgery. This organism also is involved in a significant minority of lung abscesses and cases of empy-

ema. It can also be involved in some severe soft tissue infections (along with other anaerobes and aerobes) such as Fournier's gangrene.

REFERENCES

Onderdonk, A. B., J. G. Bartlett, T. Louie, N. Sullivan-Seigler, and S. L. Gorbach. 1976. Microbial synergy in experimental intra-abdominal abscess. *Infect. Immun.* **13**:22–26.

Onderdonk, A. B., D. L. Kasper, R. L. Cisneros, and J. G. Bartlett. 1977. The capsular polysaccharide of *Bacteroides fragilis* as a virulence factor: comparison of the pathogenic potential of encapsulated and unencapsulated strains. *J. Infect. Dis.* **136**:82–89.

This 63-year-old alcoholic was taken to the emergency room of an outside hospital with obvious gangrene of both feet. He was stuporous. During that evening, he had a seizure and was treated with phenytoin and barbiturates. By the night of transfer he was noted to have opisthotonic posturing and to have developed increasing rigor, respiratory distress, and unresponsiveness. On examination, he had a temperature of 41.7°C rectally, a blood pressure of 70/30 mmHg, a heart rate of 110 beats/min, and a respiratory rate of 40/min. Examination was notable for marked trismus. The neck was stiff and hyper-extended. Necrotic, blackened areas were present over both feet and several draining ulcers were noted on the heels and toes. Neurologically the patient responded to deep pain with a grimace. On the basis of these findings, specific therapy, in addition to supportive care, was initiated, and the patient ultimately recovered.

1. What is the etiology of his infection? What virulence factor produced by the etiologic agent of his infection was responsible for his trismus?

2. How did this patient become infected with this organism? What was the role of his gangrenous feet in the development of this infection?

3. What was the specific therapy used to treat this infection?

4. How might this infection have been prevented?

DISCUSSION

1. This patient had tetanus, which is caused by *Clostridium tetani*. *C. tetani* is a strictly anaerobic, sporeforming, gram-positive rod. Because of its exquisite sensitivity to oxygen it is very difficult to recover from clinical specimens, so this diagnosis is generally made on the basis of clinical findings. The organism produces a protein exotoxin, tetanospasmin. Tetanospasmin is a neurotoxin which acts to block neurotransmitter release from inhibitory neurons. This suppression of inhibitory nerve function results in an increased activation of nerves innervating muscles (such as the masseter), causing muscle spasm.

2. *C. tetani* is typically found as spores in soil. It has a worldwide distribution. These spores can enter wounds, and if the oxidation-reduction potential (a measure of how anaerobic an environment is) is low enough, i.e., anaerobic enough, the spores will germinate and the organism can begin to grow and produce toxin in the wound. Gangrenous tissues create an ideal environment for *C. tetani* to grow. These tissues are composed of devitalized (dead) tissue with compromised blood flow, which creates a very low oxidation potential at that site. If these tissues become contaminated by soil, infection with *C. tetani* may ensue. Since many alcoholics have extremely poor personal hygiene, soil contamination of the feet is certainly very feasible.

3. Two strategies are required. The patient will require supportive therapy, particularly cleansing of the wound and ventilatory assistance. The other strategy is to use human tetanus immune globulin (TIG). This product, unlike the horse product used for diphtheria (see case 9), will not cause anaphylaxis or serum sickness. This patient received human TIG and recovered.

4. The same strategy used for prevention of diphtheria (see case 9) is also operative for tetanus. A series of four primary immunizations starting at 2 months of age followed by appropriate booster vaccinations, in adults at 10-year intervals, is highly effective in preventing tetanus. Nevertheless, 50 to 100 cases of tetanus are reported to the Centers for Disease Control annually. By contrast, approximately 3 cases of diphtheria are reported annually. The majority of tetanus cases are seen in individuals older than 60 years and it is speculated that these individuals have not received booster immunization. Public health officials are confident that tetanus levels could be reduced to the level seen with diphtheria if the geriatric population received booster vaccinations.

REFERENCES

Schofield, F. 1986. Selective primary health care: strategies for control of disease in the developing world. XXII. Tetanus: a preventable problem. *Rev. Infect. Dis.* **8:**144–156.

Weinstein, L. 1973. Tetanus. *N. Engl. J. Med.* **289:**1293–1296.

The patient was an 85-year-old female with an advanced squamous cell carcinoma of the bladder, who was admitted for treatment of a presumed cellulitis of her right lower leg. On examination, the patient appeared chronically ill. The right heel had a bluish hematoma and blister with approximately 6 by 6 cm of erythema medially. Laboratory studies on admission were notable for an elevated white blood cell count of 33,200/mm^3 with a left shift. The patient was treated with intravenous antibiotics for 2 days but her condition did not improve. She underwent a radiograph of the right ankle and foot, which demonstrated extensive gas in the soft tissues. She was taken for surgical debridement and ultimately a below-the-knee amputation. A Gram stain of the wound aspirate revealed rare polymorphonuclear leukocytes and many boxcar-shaped, gram-positive rods. (See Figure 8.) No growth was seen on aerobic cultures. The patient's condition worsened, and she died.

1. Which genus of bacteria can cause the type of infection described in this case? Several species of this genus are commonly associated with this infection. List three of them.

2. Explain the finding of gas in the soft tissues.

3. Which virulence factors play an important role in the spread of these organisms through tissue?

4. Why was it necessary to amputate her leg below the knee?

5. Explain the possible ways in which this woman could have become infected.

DISCUSSION

1 and 2. This patient has gas gangrene of her leg. This disease is most frequently associated with a group of *Clostridium* spp. which are referred to as being histotoxic. The finding on Gram stain of boxcar-shaped, gram-positive rods that do not grow aerobically is consistent with *Clostridium* spp., especially *Clostridium perfringens*. *C. perfringens* is the species of histotoxic clostridia most frequently associated with gas gangrene. This organism is a prodigious gas producer and is the most rapidly growing organism recovered from human infections. The gas seen in the tissue of this woman is a metabolic end product of metabolism of the histotoxic clostridia. Other histotoxic clostridia include *C. novyi, C. fallax, C. sordellii, C. histolyticum,* and *C. septicum.*

3. The histotoxic clostridia produce a variety of virulence factors which can degrade tissues and promote the spread of organisms throughout them. *C. perfringens* strains, for example, produce numerous virulence factors, including a lecithinase that is capable of lysing various cell types, a protease, hyaluronidase, collagenase, and various other hemolysins. The combination of virulence factors produced is strain dependent. All strains produce lecithinase (also called alpha-toxin), which appears to play a central role in pathogenesis of gas gangrene due to this organism. One of the key findings in gas gangrene is the presence of a large number of bacteria and a relative paucity of white blood cells in a Gram stain of tissue. Lecithinase can lyse white blood cells, enhancing its ability to evade the immune system and spread through tissues.

4. Gas gangrene, once established, is extremely difficult to control with only antimicrobial therapy. Because of the massive tissue damage, the affected tissue becomes devitalized, with compromise of the circulation. This compromise results in the inability of antimicrobial agents to penetrate into the infected tissue. The infection will continue its spread, especially along tissue planes, and the only way to effectively contain it is to remove the infected tissue, in this case the woman's lower leg. A serious complication of this infection is toxemia due to the alpha-toxin. This toxin can induce intravascular hemolysis, resulting in renal failure and death. The infected extremity is removed in part to prevent this ominous complication.

5. The most likely source of this organism in this woman is her own gastrointestinal tract. Clostridia are commonly found as members of the gastrointestinal tract flora and can be found colonizing the skin, especially in the perirectal region. Breaks in the skin are common in the elderly as the skin becomes more fragile with age. The clostridia can enter these breaks, producing a cellulitis. Because of her age, we would expect this patient to

have poor circulation in her extremities. Poor circulation coupled with clostridial cellulitis may result in gas gangrene, as was seen in this patient. Clostridia are commonly found in soil and may cause gas gangrene following trauma, especially when penetrating or crush injuries occur.

REFERENCES

Gorbach, S. L., and H. Thadepalli. 1985. Isolation of *Clostridium* in human infections: evaluation of 114 cases. *J. Infect. Dis.* **131:**S81–S85.

Maclennan, J. D. 1962. The histotoxic clostridial infections of man. *Bacteriol. Rev.* **26:**177–274.

CASE 31

This 39-year-old male was in his usual state of good health until mid-July, when he developed myalgias and fever. These symptoms resolved. Two weeks prior to evaluation, he developed large, erythematous, annular rashes on his right forearm, right hip, and left knee. He subsequently developed a left facial (cranial nerve VII) palsy. His history was notable only for travel to the northeastern United States (Connecticut and Rhode Island) prior to the onset of his symptoms. On physical examination, the patient was afebrile and had normal vital signs. A skin examination demonstrated the three skin lesions noted above, which had, according to the patient, faded significantly. A neurologic examination demonstrated left facial nerve weakness. The remainder of the examination was normal. Laboratory studies included a normal complete blood count. A lumbar puncture was performed. His CSF contained 78 nucleated cells/mm^3 with 88% lymphocytes and 12% monocytes. His CSF glucose level was 60 mg/dl, and the protein level was 55 mg/dl. The clinical diagnosis was confirmed serologically.

1. What do you think was the etiologic agent of his infection? Which signs and symptoms were important clues?

2. What is the significance of this patient's travel history and the time of year he was infected?

3. How does one acquire this infection?

4. Which laboratory studies are useful in establishing the diagnosis of this infection?

DISCUSSION

1. This patient has a classic presentation for Lyme disease, which is caused by the spirochete *Borrelia burgdorferi*. His constellation of symptoms, including an erythematous annular rash, meningitis with a characteristic cerebrospinal fluid examination including >50% lymphocytes, and facial palsy, are all consistent with Lyme disease. The rash is particularly helpful in establishing this diagnosis. Patients with Lyme disease have a characteristic rash referred to as erythema migrans. The rash typically has a targetlike appearance with expanding borders. Target lesions at multiple sites, as seen in this patient, are not unusual.

2. The regions in the United States in which Lyme disease is endemic are primarily the northeastern states, Minnesota, Wisconsin, and northern California. His travel history to an area of endemicity heightens the suspicion that he has Lyme disease. The peak activity of Lyme disease is seen in June to August when the *Ixodes* tick, the vector for this disease, is most actively feeding. His presentation in July further supports the diagnosis of Lyme disease.

3. *B. burgdorferi* is spread to humans primarily by ticks of the genus *Ixodes*. In the northeastern United States, the white-footed mouse appears to be the primary reservoir of *B. burgdorferi*, which is present in the bloodstream of the host. It also is the preferred host for the *Ixodes dammini* tick, the major vector for this spirochete. In other geographic locales, other *Ixodes* species act as major vectors.

   All three stages in the life cycle of the tick, i.e., larva, nymph, and adult, can feed on a human host, but only the nymph and adult stages can transmit the disease. Nymphs and adults infected after feeding on a *B. burgdorferi*-infected mouse pass the organism to humans during a blood meal, probably by regurgitating the spirochetes into the wound. Transfer of the spirochetes from the infected ticks to humans appears to require 12 to 24 h of contact. Ticks removed before that time probably do not transmit the spirochete. However, the nymph stage of the tick is extremely small (described as the size of a pencil point), so the tick bite may go unnoticed. To prevent prolonged contact with the tick, skin should be carefully examined especially when the individual has spent time in the tick's habitat. The tick is most frequently found in wooded areas but also can be found in grassy areas such as lawns.

4. This organism is fairly difficult to grow from clinical specimens and requires complex media not available in most clinical laboratories, making culture a low-yield procedure. Because of this, isolation of this organism from clinical specimens is not routinely attempted. The diagnosis is usu-

ally made on clinical grounds. Serologic tests for this organism are available, but several problems are associated with them. First, the tests are not well standardized, making them difficult to interpret. Second, the immune response may not be detectable until 4 weeks after the onset of symptoms, making diagnosis of acute disease by serology of little value. Third, cross-reactions occur between other spirochetes and *B. burgdorferi*, leading to false-positive serologic results. Fourth, in endemic areas, individuals may have serologic evidence of prior infection, complicating the interpretation of the serologic results.

Despite these difficulties, serologic testing still is the best available laboratory methodology to support the diagnosis of Lyme disease. Many institutions try to detect immunoglobulin M (IgM) antibodies to the spirochete in patients with signs and symptoms consistent with Lyme disease, usually by means of an EIA. For patients with more complicated symptoms, physicians may request a confirmatory Western immunoblot. In this test, antibodies that react with *B. burgdorferi*-specific proteins are sought. When these antibodies are present, the diagnosis is confirmed. The combination of these tests appears to be the most reliable approach to laboratory diagnosis of this disease.

REFERENCES

Buchstein, S. R., and P. Gardner. 1991. Lyme disease. *Infect. Dis. Clin. N. Am.* **5:**103-116.
Rahn, D. W., and S. E. Malawista. 1991. Lyme disease: recommendations for diagnosis and treatment. *Ann. Intern. Med.* **114:**472-491.

CASE 32

The patient was a 6-year-old female from North Carolina. She was in her usual state of good health until 10 days prior to admission, when she had a tick removed from her scalp. She developed sore throat, malaise, and a low-grade fever 8 days after tick removal. She was seen by her pediatrician when she began developing a pink, macular rash, which started on her palms and lower extremities and spread to cover her entire body. The pediatrician's diagnosis was viral exanthem. One day prior to admission, she developed purpura, emesis, diarrhea, myalgias, and increased fever. On the day of admission, she was taken to her local hospital emergency room because of mental status changes and was admitted. Her physical examination was significant for diffuse purpura; periorbital, hand, and foot edema; cool extremities with weak pulses; and hepatosplenomegaly. Her laboratory studies were significant for a Na^+ level of 125 mmol/liter, platelet count of 26,000/mm^3, WBC count of 14,900/mm^3, hemoglobin level of 8.8 g/liter, and greatly increased coagulation times. Ampicillin and chloramphenicol therapy was begun, and she was intubated and transferred to our institution; she died soon after arrival.

1. Which infectious agents are spread by ticks? Was the observation that a tick had been removed from her scalp important in this case?

2. Which condition(s) do her physical findings on admission suggest? List three organisms that can cause these types of physical findings.

3. What is the etiologic agent of this infection? Which laboratory findings are consistent with this infection?

4. Which specific test(s) is available for diagnosis of this infection?

DISCUSSION

1. Ticks are vectors for *Borrelia burgdorferi* (the agent of Lyme disease), other *Borrelia* species (which cause relapsing fever), *Francisella tularensis* (the agent of tularemia), *Babesia* spp. (the agent of babesiosis), *Rickettsia rickettsii* (the etiologic agent of Rocky Mountain spotted fever [RMSF]), and other rickettsial diseases not found in the United States. *R. rickettsii* is endemic in the state of North Carolina, with Oklahoma or North Carolina reporting the largest number of RMSF cases on a yearly basis. The incubation time after tick exposure ranges from 2 to 14 days, with a median of 7 days. Her development of symptoms 8 days after tick exposure is consistent with *R. rickettsii* infection.

2. The findings of cool extremities with weak pulses are indicative of shock. Edema is the result of increased vascular permeability, suggesting damage to endothelial cells, a well-known mechanism of *R. rickettsii*-induced pathologic changes. Purpura in the setting of septic shock indicates that the patient is suffering from disseminated intravascular coagulation (DIC). Her platelet count and coagulation times are consistent with DIC. Almost any aerobic, gram-negative organism can cause septic shock and DIC; these include *Neisseria meningitidis*, *Vibrio vulnificus*, *Pseudomonas aeruginosa*, members of the family *Enterobacteriaceae*, *Pasteurella multocida*, and *Haemophilus influenzae*. *Streptococcus pneumoniae* and *R. rickettsii* can also cause septic shock. In the southwestern United States, *Yersinia pestis* should also be considered in the differential diagnosis of patients with septic shock and DIC.

3. The most likely etiology of her infection is *R. rickettsii*, which causes Rocky Mountain spotted fever. Hyponatremia (low Na^+ level) is commonly seen in RMSF, as are low platelet counts and increased coagulation times, both of which are manifestations of DIC, an often fatal complication of this infection.

4. This organism can be detected directly in tissue biopsy specimens by using the direct fluorescent antibody technique. This technique has the advantage of being very rapid and, in skilled hands, very specific. However, its sensitivity is very much dependent on the quality of the tissue biopsy. A negative test does not rule out this diagnosis. This test is available in only a limited number of laboratories. The polymerase chain reaction has also been applied to the detection of this organism but is not yet widely available. The organism can also be isolated from blood by inoculation of guinea pigs, embryonated eggs, or tissue culture. However, cultivation of this organism is extremely dangerous and is attempted only in a few highly specialized laboratories.

Serologic tests are the most widely used diagnostic tests for detection of RMSF. In this hospital we use both a dot blot EIA test and an indirect fluorescent antibody (IFA) test. The EIA is highly specific and has very good sensitivity. False-negative results do occur, so alternative serologic tests should be available. The IFA test can be used to confirm the EIA test and also can be used as a primary diagnostic test. One of the major problems with the serologic tests is that early in the disease course, the individual may not have mounted a sufficiently strong immune response to result in a positive serologic test result. Follow-up serologic tests 1 to 4 weeks later may prove positive. In patients in whom RMSF is a distinct possibility, a negative serologic test result should not preclude the use of antimicrobial therapy since a fulminant, fatal disease course with this organism, as was seen in this case, is not unusual.

REFERENCE

Walker, D. H. 1989. Rocky Mountain spotted fever: a disease in need of microbiological concern. *Clin. Microbiol. Rev.* **2:**227–240.

CASE 33

The patient was a 42-year-old male. One week prior to admission, he had a renal biopsy because of a 20-lb (9-kg) weight gain with peripheral edema. His biopsy showed minimal changes. Therapy with prednisone and diuretics was begun. On admission, he presented with right calf pain and a syncopal episode, and he was hypotensive. He was tachypneic and had a pulse of 121 beats/min and a temperature of 38.5°C. Two blood cultures taken at admission grew an oxidase-positive, gram-negative rod on MacConkey agar; this bacterium was presumptively identified as a *Pseudomonas* sp. On the second hospital day, the organism was found to be a glucose fermenter. On learning that the oxidase-positive organism was a fermenter, we requested that it be determined whether the patient had recently eaten raw seafood. Two days prior to admission, he had celebrated his negative renal biopsy by taking his wife to dinner. During dinner, he ate raw oysters. The dinner was in the month of August.

1. Which family of bacteria is composed of oxidase-positive, glucose-fermenting, gram-negative rods?

2. How did the patient's treatment for his renal insufficiency predispose him to infection?

3. The patient's presentation was consistent with which clinical state?

4. What was the role of the patient's consumption of seafood in the development of his infection?

5. What is the etiologic agent of this infection? What is the appropriate antimicrobial therapy?

DISCUSSION

1. The major family of organisms that grow on MacConkey agar and are oxidase-positive, glucose-fermenting, gram-negative rods is the *Vibrionaceae*. This family includes the genera *Vibrio*, *Aeromonas*, and *Plesiomonas*, all of which are associated with gastrointestinal diseases. Systemic infections, as was seen in this case, are unusual with these organisms.

2. Prednisone is a corticosteroid used to treat inflammatory processes which may have been occurring in the kidneys of this patient. Patients receiving this immunosuppressive therapy are believed to be at increased risk for infections.

3. Rapid respiration and pulse rates and very low blood pressure are consistent with septic shock.

4. Halophilic vibrios have been recovered from raw oysters and clams from water which meets federally mandated guidelines for fecal contamination. The etiologic agent in this case, *Vibrio vulnificus*, has been isolated from raw oysters. Most individuals can consume contaminated raw oysters with impunity. This organism causes septicemia almost exclusively in individuals with hepatic cirrhosis or underlying immunocompromised states. In this case, we speculate that prednisone therapy predisposed this individual to infection.

    Cases of systemic *V. vulnificus* infection are seen most commonly in months when the temperature of the water from which raw seafood is harvested is highest. Cases occur most frequently between June and October. It is speculated that the number of vibrios increases as the water temperature rises and that therefore the level of seafood contamination also increases.

5. This patient had *V. vulnificus* septicemia. Rapid initiation of appropriate antimicrobial therapy for this infection is critical. In a case review by Klontz et al., the longer the delay in the initiation of antimicrobial therapy, the higher the mortality. Mortality was 33% if antimicrobial agents were given within the first 24 h and 100% if they were delayed by 72 h. The therapy of choice is tetracycline. This patient received a broad-spectrum cephalosporin, ceftriaxone, and had an uneventful recovery.

REFERENCE

Klontz, K. C., S. Lieb, M. Schreiber, H. T. Janowski, L. M. Baldy, and R. A. Gunn. 1988. Syndromes of *Vibrio vulnificus* infections. *Ann. Intern. Med.* **109**:318–323.

CASE 34

The patient, a 16-year-old female, was well until 2 days prior to admission, when she had fever to 39.9°C and vomiting. On the morning of admission, she had loose stools, continued fever, and vomiting. She was seen by an outside physician, who noted that she was hypotensive (blood pressure, 76/48 mmHg) with a heart rate of 120 beats/min and a temperature of 38°C. She had an erythematous rash. Blood, throat, and vaginal specimens were sent for culture; the patient was given intravenous fluids and intravenous antibiotics and transported to our hospital for admission to the pediatric intensive care unit. Laboratory studies indicated abnormal liver (albumin, 2.9 g/liter; aspartate aminotransferase [AST], 76 U/liter; alanine aminotransferase [ALT], 95 U/liter) and renal (creatinine, 2.8 mg/dl) functions and WBC count of 14,100/mm^3 with 78% neutrophils and 18% band forms. The patient began her menstrual period 4 days prior to admission and uses tampons.

1. The patient's symptoms are most representative of which syndrome?

2. The vaginal culture was positive for a heavy growth of catalase-positive, gram-positive cocci. Which organism would you expect this to be?

3. Which virulence factor does this organism produce that is believed to be responsible for the signs and symptoms seen in this patient?

4. What is the significance of tampon use in this patient?

DISCUSSION

1. This patient has staphylococcal toxic shock syndrome (TSS). This syndrome is characterized by erythema, diarrhea, and low blood pressure. All these signs were seen in this patient. This syndrome is most commonly seen in menstruating women between 15 and 25 years of age. However, it should be emphasized that this is not a disease just of menstruating women. In fact, the first case of this disease was recognized in an 8-year-old boy. Cases occur in men but are frequently misdiagnosed because of the misconception that toxic shock syndrome is a disease only of women. For example, we recently saw a 28-year-old man who had poison ivy superinfected with *Staphylococcus aureus*. The physician caring for him became suspicious of toxic shock syndrome on noting a sudden drop in blood pressure and some diarrhea. A culture from his skin lesions was positive for an *S. aureus* isolate which produced toxic shock syndrome toxin 1 (TSST-1).

2 and 3. The organism is likely to be *S. aureus*. The finding of a heavy growth of *S. aureus* is supportive but does not prove the diagnosis of toxic shock syndrome. First, *S. aureus* is part of the normal vaginal flora in 8 to 10% of women, and although heavy vaginal growth of *S. aureus* would be highly unusual, it is possible. Second, to prove that this isolate is the etiologic agent of toxic shock syndrome, it should be demonstrated that the isolate produced TSST-1. This isolate was shown to produce this virulence factor. In animal models this toxin reproduces at least some of the clinical characteristics of this disease as seen in humans. The manner by which TSST-1 induces this disease is controversial.

4. One of the key observations in the initial epidemic of TSS was that the disease was most severe in women who used superabsorbent tampons. When the association between superabsorbent tampons and TSS became clear, this product was withdrawn from the U.S. marketplace. With this suspension in sales came a marked decrease in the number of cases of TSS. Sporadic cases continue to occur, most commonly in menstruating women who use tampons.

REFERENCES

Schlievert, P. M., K. N. Shauds, B. B. Dan, G. P. Schmid, and R. D. Nishimura. 1981. Identification and characterization of an exotoxin from *Staphylococcus aureus* associated with toxic-shock syndrome. *J. Infect. Dis.* **143**:509–516.

Todd, J., M. Fishaut, F. Kapral, and T. Welch. 1978. Toxic shock syndrome associated with phage-group-1 staphylococci. *Lancet* **ii**:1116–1118.

Table 1. Medically important bacteria

Aerobic, gram-positive cocci	**Aerobic, gram-positive rods**
Coagulase-negative staphylococci	*Bacillus anthracis*
Enterococcus spp.	*Bacillus cereus*
Group C and G streptococci	*Corynebacterium diphtheriae*
Staphylococcus aureus	Diphtheroids
Streptococcus agalactiae (group B)	*Lactobacillus* spp.
Streptococcus bovis (group D)	*Listeria monocytogenes*
Streptococcus pneumoniae	*Nocardia* spp.
Streptococcus pyogenes (group A)	*Rhodococcus equi*
Viridans streptococci	
Aerobic, gram-negative cocci	**Anaerobic, gram-negative rods**
Moraxella catarrhalis	*Bacteroides fragilis*
Neisseria gonorrhoeae	*Bacteroides* spp.
Neisseria meningitidis	*Fusobacterium nucleatum*
	Fusobacterium spp.
Fastidious aerobic, gram-negative rods	**Anaerobic, gram-positive rods**
Actinobacillus actinomycetemcomitans	*Actinomyces* sp.
Bordetella pertussis	*Clostridium botulinum*
Brucella abortus	*Clostridium difficile*
Brucella canis	*Clostridium fallax*
Brucella melitensis	*Clostridium histolyticum*
Brucella suis	*Clostridium novyi*
Campylobacter fetus	*Clostridium perfringens*
Campylobacter jejuni	*Clostridium septicum*
Capnocytophaga sp.	*Clostridium tetani*
Cardiobacterium hominis	
Eikenella corrodens	
Francisella tularensis	
Haemophilus aphrophilus	
Haemophilus ducreyi	
Haemophilus influenzae	
Haemophilus parainfluenzae	
Helicobacter pylori	
Kingella kingii	
Legionella pneumophila	
Pasteurella multocida	

(Continued)

Table 1. *(continued)*

Enterobacteriaceae (glucose-fermenting, gram-negative rods)	Bacteria which cannot be Gram stained
Citrobacter spp.	*Borrelia burgdorferi*
Enterobacter spp.	*Chlamydia psittaci*
Escherichia coli	*Chlamydia trachomatis*
Klebsiella pneumoniae	*Coxiella burnetii*
Proteus spp.	*Mycobacterium avium complex*
Salmonella enteriditis	*Mycobacterium tuberculosis*
Salmonella typhi	*Rickettsia rickettsii*
Serratia marcescens	*Treponema pallidum*
Shigella dysenteriae	
Shigella flexneri	Glucose-nonfermenting, gram-negative rods
Shigella sonnei	*Acinetobacter* spp.
Yersinia enterocolitica	*Flavobacterium meningosepticum*
Yersinia pestis	*Pseudomonas aeruginosa*
	Pseudomonas cepacia
Oxidase-positive, glucose-fermenting gram-negative rods	*Xanthomonas maltophilia*
Aeromonas spp.	
Plesiomonas shigelloides	
Vibrio cholerae	
Vibrio parahaemolyticus	
Vibrio vulnificus	

MYCOLOGY AND PARASITOLOGY

Infections due to various fungi, protozoans, and worms are often poorly understood by medical students. This group of pathogens is, too often, believed to be infrequently encountered and of limited clinical importance. This attitude has never been particularly accurate, but forces in our society have made it more and more fallacious. Protection from both groups of organisms is dependent on the functioning of the cell-mediated arm of our immune system. Both AIDS and the use of powerful immunosuppressive agents have created populations which not only are at increased risk for infections with these agents but have suffered significant morbidity and mortality from them.

Jet travel has made it possible for ever greater numbers of people to visit or emigrate from areas endemic for parasitic infections not present in the United States. Physicians need a better grasp of geographical medicine and the parasitic infections encountered in various regions of the world. The purpose of this section is to present cases due to fungi and parasites so that students can gain confidence in recognizing clinical situations in which these organisms may be important.

This 4-year-old boy was taken by his mother to the dermatology clinic for evaluation of a 2-month history of a slowly growing "bump" on the back of his head. Examination revealed a happy, alert child in no distress. A raised, scaling lesion 3.5 cm in diameter with a few pinpoint pustules was present on the posterior scalp. A potassium hydroxide preparation of material from the lesion was negative. A Wood's lamp examination of the scalp did not demonstrate significant fluorescence. A fungal culture of material from the lesion was positive for a fungus with numerous microconidia; macroconidia were not seen.

1. This patient has a scalp infection with what type of organism? Which genera cause these infections?

2. How does the microscopic appearance help in assigning this fungus to a genus?

3. Other than the scalp, where does infection with this type of fungus take place?

4. Where in nature are these agents found?

5. How are these types of infections treated?

DISCUSSION

1. This patient had an infection with a dermatophyte. The dermatophytes are molds that cause superficial infections of the skin, nails, and hair. Three genera of dermatophytes are pathogenic for humans: *Trichophyton*, *Microsporum*, and *Epidermophyton*.

2. The presence of many microconidia indicates this mold is probably in the genus *Trichophyton*. This isolate was ultimately identified as *Trichophyton tonsurans*. Members of the genus *Microsporum* are identified as such by the presence of multiseptate lancet-shaped macroconidia with few or absent microconidia. *Epidermophyton* (which contains only one species, *Epidermophyton floccosum*) cultures demonstrate large, club-shaped macroconidia and does not produce microconidia.

   The Wood's lamp was used in the evaluation of this patient because in scalp infections caused by some *Microsporum* species the hairs will fluoresce green when examined under ultraviolet light.

3. *Trichophyton* infections can occur in any keratinized tissue including skin, hair, and nails; *Microsporum* species usually infect the hair and skin and *E. floccosum* infects primarily the skin and nails. These organisms are very rarely invasive, causing primarily superficial infections. The word "tinea" (worm) is used to describe the location of the infection. Tinea capitis is an infection of the head, tinea cruris is an infection of the groin (jock itch), and tinea pedis is an infection of the foot (athlete's foot).

   Typically an annular scaling rash with a raised margin is present. The margin or edge (not the center) of such a lesion is the appropriate site for examination and culture because that is the site in the lesion where the organism is growing.

4. These infections are acquired from soil (often in areas where keratinized debris is accumulated), animals (for example, *Microsporum canis* is found on dogs and cats), and other humans. Outbreaks of tinea capitis frequently occur in young children, who contract the organism from classmates.

5. Topical therapy is used in many cases. Keeping the groin and the feet dry following exercise and showers will control or prevent most cases of jock itch and athlete's foot. Nail and hair infections are treated with oral antifungal agents such as ketoconazole and griseofulvin. Infected fingernails and toenails require prolonged therapy, and relapse is common.

REFERENCE

Leyden, J. J., and A. M. Kligman. 1978. Interdigital athlete's foot, the interaction of dermatophytes and resident bacteria. *Arch. Dermatol.* **114:**1466–1472.

This 71-year-old woman was admitted with a recurrence of her poorly differentiated squamous cell carcinoma of the cervix. She underwent extensive gynecologic surgery (excision of the organs of the anterior pelvis) and was maintained postoperatively on broad-spectrum intravenous antibiotics. The patient had a central venous catheter placed on the day of the surgery.

Beginning 3 days postoperatively, the patient had temperatures of 38.0 to 38.5°C, which persisted without a clear source. On day 8 postoperatively, she had a temperature of 39.2°C. Cultures of blood and of the tip of the central line both grew an agent that was ovoid and reproduced by budding. (See Figure 9.)

1. What is the differential diagnosis of this patient's infecting organism?

2. The organism was subsequently shown to form germ tubes. What is the organism?

3. Is this organism part of normal flora in humans?

4. How did treatment with broad-spectrum antibiotics predispose this patient to infection with this organism?

5. The same organism was present in a positive culture of blood and in a culture of the central venous catheter tip. What does this suggest in terms of the portal of entry of the organism causing the infection?

DISCUSSION

1. The presence of ovoid yeast cells that reproduce by budding is consistent with a *Candida* species (such as *Candida albicans, C. tropicalis, C. parapsilosis, C. lusitaniae, C. krusei,* and *C. guilliermondii*) or with *Torulopsis* (formerly classified as *Candida*) *glabrata. Histoplasma capsulatum* is also often ovoid and may demonstrate budding, but is not confused with *Candida* species because of its smaller size. In addition, it grows more slowly than do *Candida* species. Although isolates of *Cryptococcus neoformans* typically demonstrate round yeast cells, this species should be considered when a yeast is isolated from a blood or cerebrospinal fluid sample.

2. *C. albicans* can be differentiated from other *Candida* species on the basis of its ability to form germ tubes. This test is done by incubating suspected *Candida*-like isolates in human or animal serum for 1 to 2 h and examining the organisms microscopically for germ tube formation. Most but not all *C. albicans* isolates are germ tube positive. The germ tube test is an excellent presumptive test for identification of *C. albicans. Candida* species which are germ tube negative are identified by using carbohydrate utilization and biochemical tests.

3. *Candida* species are a part of the normal flora of the skin, gastrointestinal tract, oropharynx, and vagina.

4. Treatment of patients with broad-spectrum antibacterial agents may allow the growth of yeasts in situations in which they would otherwise be inhibited by the normal bacterial flora. For example, candidal vaginitis is often associated with the prior use of a broad-spectrum antibiotic. The normal bacterial flora may compete with *Candida* species for nutrients. Alternatively, the normal flora may create an unfavorable environment for *Candida* species. When the normal flora is eliminated, the *Candida* species is no longer inhibited and overgrowth of the yeast may occur.

    In recent years mucocutaneous candidiasis (often including involvement of the esophagus) has been caused by immunosuppression due to infection with the human immunodeficiency virus (HIV). Unexplained oral thrush is one clue to the presence of an HIV infection.

5. Since *C. albicans* does not normally invade the bloodstream, a breakdown of host defenses must occur to allow a blood-borne infection (candidemia). The two most important defenses in this regard are (i) the presence of an intact barrier (skin) between the blood vessels and the outside and (ii) the presence of an adequate number of functioning neutrophils. With regard to the first defense, since *Candida* species may be present on the skin, intravenous drug users and patients with intravenous devices (such

as this patient) are at increased risk of blood-borne infection. Patients lacking the second defense often have cancer and have been left with few neutrophils as a result of chemotherapy. The presence of the same organism in blood and on the central venous catheter tip suggests that this patient may have become infected via the breach in the integrity of the skin at the site of the central line insertion. The blood would then be seeded from the central line. A less likely possibility is that the patient had candidemia from another source and that the central venous catheter was seeded from the blood-borne infection.

REFERENCES

Bonacini, M., T. Young, and L. Laine. 1991. The causes of esophageal symptoms in human immunodeficiency virus infection. A prospective study of 110 patients. *Arch. Intern. Med.* **151:**1567–1572.

Komshian, S. V., A. K. Uwaydah, J. D. Sopel, and L. R. Crane. 1989. Fungemia caused by *Candida* species and *Torulopsis glabrata* in the hospitalized patient: frequency, characteristics, and evaluation of factors influencing outcome. *Rev. Infect. Dis.* **11:**379–390.

This 37-year-old man was admitted to the hospital with an increased white blood cell count and a peripheral smear consistent with acute leukemia. A bone marrow biopsy found 70 to 80% blast forms diagnostic of acute myelomonocytic leukemia. The patient underwent induction chemotherapy. Following the chemotherapy, a repeat bone marrow biopsy again demonstrated blast forms. He therefore underwent a second round of induction chemotherapy, after which he became profoundly neutropenic (with fewer than 100 neutrophils/mm^3) and developed fevers without a clear source. Broad-spectrum antibiotic therapy was begun, but the fevers persisted. Empirical intravenous amphotericin B therapy was begun, and a subsequent chest radiograph revealed new bilateral fluffy pulmonary infiltrates. A bronchoscopy with biopsy was performed; it demonstrated septate hyphae with acute-angle branching. (See Figure 10.)

1. What is the differential diagnosis of pulmonary infiltrates in a leukemic patient?

2. Which fungus was seen on the specimen from bronchoscopy? Why was biopsy and not lavage necessary to make this diagnosis?

3. Would blood cultures have been useful in helping to make this diagnosis? Explain your answer.

4. Where in nature is this fungus found?

5. What predisposed this patient to this infection?

6. What other types of infections are caused by this fungus?

DISCUSSION

1. Infectious causes of pulmonary infiltrates in leukemic patients include bacterial (especially gram-negative rods and *Staphylococcus aureus*), fungal (including *Aspergillus* species, zygomycetes, *Cryptococcus neoformans*, and *Candida* species), viral (including cytomegalovirus), and parasitic (such as *Pneumocystis carinii*) organisms. Noninfectious causes of pulmonary infiltrates in these patients include bleeding into the lung and leukemic infiltrates.

2. The presence of septate hyphae (3 to 4 μm in diameter) with acute-angle branching is consistent with the presence of an *Aspergillus* species. The species cannot be determined by the morphologic appearance of the fungus from a tissue specimen; culture is required. On culture, the isolate in this case was *Aspergillus flavus*. Other clinically significant species include *A. fumigatus* and *A. niger*. This patient had invasive aspergillosis. In this disease, the organism actually grows into the tissue and often is not found superficially in the airway. Therefore lavage is not sufficient and a tissue sample is needed to make this diagnosis.

3. Because they are almost never positive in patients with invasive aspergillosis, blood cultures have little diagnostic value. In patients with invasive aspergillosis, the organism has a predilection for invading endothelial cells and, as a result, is rarely present in the bloodstream. In invasive disease, infection of the endothelial cells can lead to thrombosis and infarction of the infected vessels and of the tissue supplied by those vessels.

4. *Aspergillus* species can be isolated from grains, hay, decaying vegetable matter, soil, and plants. Aflatoxin B_1, a potent carcinogen that has been linked to hepatocellular carcinoma, is produced by strains of *A. flavus* on improperly stored grains and nuts. *Aspergillus* spores are present in the air. Therefore, humans are constantly exposed to (and breathe) spores of these organisms. Because of the constant exposure to these spores, people may become colonized by *Aspergillus* species without being infected and so a positive culture for an *Aspergillus* species may not be clinically significant.

5. This patient had neutropenia, a dramatically decreased number of neutrophils in his peripheral blood. This condition predisposes to invasive infections not only by bacteria but also by fungi including *Aspergillus* species. The risk of infection by fungi is related to both the severity and duration of the neutropenia. This patient not only had very few neutrophils (sometimes none were detected) but he also was neutropenic for a prolonged period. Despite treatment with intravenous amphotericin B, many leuke-

mic patients succumb to this infection. In this case, the patient's neutrophil count began to rise and he survived the infection.

6. In addition to invasive lung infection, *Aspergillus* species can cause pulmonary mycetoma (a "fungus ball" which often forms in a preexisting pulmonary cavity), allergic bronchopulmonary aspergillosis (in patients with preexisting chronic lung disease), and infections of the external ear, nasal sinuses, eyes (following corneal trauma), brain, and heart valves.

REFERENCES

Rinaldi, M. G. 1988. Aspergillosis, p. 559–572. *In* A. Balows, W. J. Hausler, Jr., M. Ohashi, and A. Turano (ed.), *Laboratory Diagnosis of Infectious Diseases: Principles and Practice*, vol. I. *Bacterial, Mycotic and Parasitic Diseases*. Springer-Verlag, New York.

Young, R.C., J. E. Bennett, C. L. Vogel, P. P. Carbone, and V. DeVita. 1970. Aspergillosis: the spectrum of the disease in 98 patients. *Medicine* 49:147–173.

This 62-year-old man presented with a 4-day history of left eye swelling and left frontal headache. He also had noted the progression of left ptosis over the 4 days. He had an unremarkable medical history, although his family history was strongly positive for diabetes mellitus. On examination, the patient was febrile to 38.1°C and had complete left ptosis. Laboratory studies were notable for an elevated white blood cell count of 17,900/mm^3 with 14,400 neutrophils/mm^3 and an elevated blood glucose level of 484 mg/dl, indicating that he is a diabetic. A CT scan of the sinuses and orbits was notable for fluid in both ethmoid sinuses and inflammatory changes lateral to the left medial rectus muscle. The patient underwent surgery (a left external ethmoidectomy). A KOH preparation of the material from the left ethmoid sinus obtained at the time of surgery demonstrated broad, aseptate hyphae with right-angle branching. (See Figure 11.)

1. Which organisms are consistent with these histologic findings?

2. Where are these organisms found in nature?

3. Which clinical conditions are associated with invasive infections with these organisms?

4. How is this infection managed? What is the prognosis for this patient?

DISCUSSION

1. The presence of broad, aseptate or sparsely septate hyphae with right-angle branching is diagnostic of an agent of zygomycosis. This includes infections with molds from the genera *Mucor, Rhizopus, Rhizomucor, Absidia,* and *Cunninghamella.* In a section from clinical material these organisms are indistinguishable. They can be differentiated from *Aspergillus* species in clinical materials since *Aspergillus* species have acute-angle branching (instead of right-angle branching as with agents of zygomycosis), frequent septations, and thin hyphae. Zygomycotic infections are extremely aggressive and frequently fatal. They represent a true medical (and surgical) emergency and differentiation from *Aspergillus* species can be crucial. Culture results showed that this patient was infected with a *Rhizopus* species.

2. The agents of zygomycosis are commonly found in the environment on fruit and bread and in soil. In fact, sterile bread devoid of preservatives (which may prevent the growth of zygomycetes) can be used as a sporulation medium for these organisms.

3. Zygomycosis is associated with several clinical conditions. Rhinocerebral zygomycosis is associated with diabetes mellitus (as with this patient), particularly with acidosis, and occurs in patients with leukemia. When there is pulmonary involvement, leukemia and lymphoma (with neutropenia) are common underlying conditions, although it may occur with diabetes as well. The skin may be infected in burn patients and, rarely, in diabetic patients. The central nervous system may be involved via direct extension from the sinuses. Pathologically, the fungus directly invades blood vessels, causing thrombosis of the blood vessels and infarction of the area that normally receives its arterial blood supply via the invaded vessel. In some cases disseminated infection can occur.

4. Since the disease, when untreated, runs a progressive and fatal course, early recognition and a high degree of suspicion are necessary. It was the suspicion of zygomycosis that caused the surgeon in this case to obtain a frozen section intraoperatively, a procedure in which the pathologist examines the tissue as rapidly as possible (without the standard techniques used to fix tissue) while the patient is still in the operating room. Often multiple frozen sections are examined during surgery. Debridement of the infected area will continue until a frozen section is obtained in which the organisms are no longer seen. Treatment includes both aggressive surgical removal of infected and necrotic tissue and antifungal therapy (intravenous amphotericin B).

REFERENCE

Parfrey, N. A. 1986. Improved diagnosis and prognosis of mucormycosis: a clinico-pathologic study of 33 cases. *Medicine* **65:**113–123.

This 35-year-old man with a history of intravenous drug use was admitted for evaluation of a productive cough, severe headache, skin lesions, nausea, vomiting, and diarrhea. Multiple cultures were obtained including cerebrospinal fluid (CSF). The CSF examination revealed a glucose level of 56 mg/dl, a protein level of 42 mg/dl, an erythrocyte (RBC) count of 5,940/mm^3, and 7 white blood cells/mm^3 (68% neutrophils, 30% lymphocytes, 1% monocytes, and 1% eosinophils). Cultures of blood, CSF, sputum, and the skin biopsy specimen were all positive for the same organism. A serologic examination was subsequently positive for antibodies to HIV-1.

1. How would you characterize the lumbar puncture done on this individual? Are these results surprising in light of the culture findings?

2. The organism cultured from the patient, when viewed under the microscope, appeared to be round with small buds connected to the larger cell via a narrow connection. When it was viewed under the microscope with India ink, the presence of a refractile capsule was noted. What is this organism?

3. In addition to culture, what other method can be used to diagnose infection with this organism? If this test was repeated several weeks after the beginning of therapy, what might the results be?

4. This patient is at risk for this infection as a result of what immunologic defect?

5. Do persons with a normal immune system become infected with this agent?

DISCUSSION

1. The lumbar puncture was traumatic; i.e., the ratio of RBC to leukocytes (WBC) is approximately 850:1, which would be a normal ratio in blood. The white blood cell differential is consistent with a "normal" differential in peripheral blood. The CSF glucose and protein levels also are within normal limits. This is not a surprising finding. Many HIV-infected individuals who develop cryptococcal meningitis have normal CSF parameters despite the presence of this organism in CSF. In contrast, in patients who are not infected with HIV, increased CSF protein levels and decreased CSF glucose levels are often seen in cases of cryptococcal meningitis.

2. *Cryptococcus neoformans* is a yeast which frequently produces a polysaccharide capsule. The capsule has been shown to protect this organism from phagocytosis. One key characteristic of this organism used to identify it in the laboratory is its ability to rapidly hydrolyze urea owing to the production of a potent urease.

3. Capsular polysaccharide antigen can be detected in both serum and CSF. Two methodologies for this detection are available, a latex agglutination test and an enzyme immunosorbent assay (EIA). Antigen detection is much more sensitive than direct examination of CSF for encapsulated organisms by using India ink or Gram stain. In HIV-infected individuals with cryptococcal meningitis, the antigen may persist in CSF for the entire life of the individual and may never be cleared, despite otherwise adequate antifungal therapy. In addition, the organisms may still be able to be visualized by direct examination even though they may no longer be viable. Capsule-deficient *C. neoformans* cells are also seen in HIV-infected individuals. These patients have negative or very low antigen titer results.

4. Most individuals at risk for developing systemic cryptococcal disease have deficits in their cell-mediated immunity. Specifically, HIV-positive individuals have reduced numbers of T-helper cells, putting them at increased risk for infection with this organism.

5. Asymptomatic infection, most likely pulmonary, is frequent. The organism is ubiquitous in nature and can be found in high concentrations in bird droppings, especially those of pigeons. Symptomatic infections, especially meningitis, occur in immunocompetent hosts but are unusual.

REFERENCES

Bennett, J. E., W. E. Dismukes, R. J. Duma, G. Medoff, M. A. Sande, H. Gallis, J. Leonard, B. T. Fields, M. Bradshaw, H. Haywood, Z. A. McGee, T. R. Cate, C. G. Cobbs, J. F. Warner, and D. W. Alling. 1979. A comparison of amphotericin B alone and combined with flucytosine in the treatment of cryptococcal meningitis. *N. Engl. J. Med.* **301**:126–131.

Diamond, R. D., and J. E. Bennett. 1974. Prognostic factors in cryptococcal meningitis. A study of 111 cases. *Ann. Intern. Med.* **80**:176–181.

Kovacs, J. A., A. A. Kovacs, M. Polis, W. C. Wright, V. J. Gill, C. U. Tuazon, E. P. Gelmann, H. C. Lane, R. Longfield, G. Overturf, A. M. Macher, A. S. Fauci, J. E. Parrillo, J. E. Bennett, and H. Masur. 1985. Cryptococcus in the acquired immunodeficiency syndrome. *Ann. Intern. Med.* **103**:533–538.

CASE 40

This 72-year-old woman with no history of tobacco use was admitted for evaluation of a right upper lobe lung mass. Five months prior to admission, the patient developed a fever and persistent cough productive of white sputum with slight hemoptysis. She was treated with an oral antibiotic. Three months prior to admission, a chest radiograph revealed a masslike lesion in the right upper lung anteriorly, near the chest wall. She denied any chest pain, dyspnea on exertion, or history of tuberculosis. A purified protein derivative (PPD) skin test was nonreactive. A bronchoscopy performed 2 months prior to admission did not reveal any endobronchial lesion, and a cytologic examination was negative for cancer. In the month of admission, a repeat chest radiograph revealed that the density in the right lung had increased in size since the previous radiograph.

The patient was admitted to the hospital, where she underwent a right thoracotomy. A frozen section of lung tissue from the lesion demonstrated granulomatous inflammation. On the basis of this result, no additional lung material was resected. Gomori methenamine silver stain of the lung tissue demonstrated ovoid yeast cells (1.5 to 2.0 by 3.0 to 3.5 μm) that were diagnostic. Subsequent culture confirmed the diagnosis.

1. What is the differential diagnosis of the patient's lung mass?

2. What was the etiologic agent of this patient's pulmonary process?

3. In which areas of the United States is this disease endemic? Where in nature is the organism found?

4. What is the portal of entry in infection with this organism? Does infection spread from this site? If so, to which organs?

5. Clinically, how does the immunosuppression in patients with AIDS cause this disease to present?

6. How is this disease treated?

DISCUSSION

1. Lung masses are caused by both noninfectious processes (such as malignant and benign tumors) and chronic infections with slowly growing organisms such as fungi (including *Blastomyces dermatitidis*, *Coccidioides immitis*, and *Histoplasma capsulatum*), mycobacteria (including *Mycobacterium tuberculosis*), and other bacteria such as *Actinomyces* and *Nocardia* spp.

2. The presence of oval to round yeast cells (some of which may have buds) that are 2 to 5 μm in size is consistent with infection with *H. capsulatum*. In histologic section this fungus can best be visualized by using the methenamine-silver stain. Wright stain of bone marrow specimens may also detect it.

   H. capsulatum is dimorphic; that is, it exists in a mold form at 25 to 30°C and as a yeast at body temperature. Other dimorphic fungi include the pathogens *B. dermatitidis*, *Sporothrix schenckii*, *C. immitis*, and *Paracoccidioides brasiliensis*. In general, the dimorphic fungi grow slowly in culture. It may take up to a month of incubation to recover *H. capsulatum* from a clinical specimen.

3. Histoplasmosis is endemic in the Ohio, Mississippi, and Missouri River valleys. Although birds are not infected with this organism, soil that is rich in bird droppings or bat guano (near chicken coops, pigeon roosts, caves, starling roosts, etc.) is a rich nutrient source for this organism and often contains it.

4. Infection is initiated by the inhalation of airborne microconidia. Activities such as cleaning chicken coops or disrupting soil (particularly on windy days) may be associated with inhalation of the spores. Although the vast majority of infections are self-limited and asymptomatic, infection may result in acute pulmonary histoplasmosis which, in most cases, requires no treatment. As with tuberculosis, infection may cause a chronic pulmonary infection. It may also progress to involve local lymph nodes, the mediastinum, pleura, or pericardium. Infection may spread hematogenously to any organ in the body. In patients living in endemic areas, the radiographic finding of calcifications in the spleen is often evidence of prior, frequently asymptomatic disease. Occasionally patients with no identifiable immune deficiency develop disseminated (and life-threatening) disease.

5. In patients with an impaired cell-mediated immunity, such as patients with AIDS, disseminated disease may occur. Fever and weight loss, common in patients with AIDS, may exist. An overwhelming infection may occur as well. Other causes of immunosuppression, such as corticosteroid therapy, may also prevent the patient's immune system from controlling

the infection. A detailed travel history must be obtained, since disease may develop even years after the patient has left an area of endemicity.

6. Like another endemic dimorphic fungus, *C. immitis*, acute infection with *H. capsulatum* usually requires no treatment. Patients with disseminated disease require antifungal therapy with either oral ketoconazole or, in immunosuppressed patients and those with meningitis or endocarditis, intravenous amphotericin B.

REFERENCES

Edwards, L. B., F. A. Acquaviva, V. T. Livesay, F. W. Cross, and C. E. Palmer. 1969. An atlas of sensitivity to tuberculin, PPD-B, and histoplasmin in the United States. *Am. Rev. Respir. Dis.* **99**(Suppl.):1–132.

Goodwin, R. A., J. E. Loyd, and R. M. DesPrez. 1981. Histoplasmosis in normal hosts. *Medicine* **60**:231–266.

Johnson, P. C., N. Khardori, A. F. Najjar, F. Butt, P. W. A. Mansell, and G. A. Sarosi. 1988. Progressive disseminated histoplasmosis in patients with acquired immunodeficiency syndrome. *Am. J. Med.* **85**:152–158.

This 38-year-old North Carolina man was in good health until 2 months prior to admission, when he developed a low-grade fever, myalgias, and a nonproductive cough. He was given oral erythromycin by his local physician. After 2 weeks of therapy, his condition had not improved. A chest radiograph demonstrated "right middle lobe air space disease," and therapy with oral ampicillin was begun. Over the next month, his condition worsened. He noted daily fevers, chills, night sweats, and a 7-kg weight loss. One month prior to admission, a chest radiograph demonstrated consolidation of the right middle lobe. A PPD skin test was negative with positive controls, and an oral antibacterial agent was given. The patient's symptoms continued, and he was admitted to the hospital.

The patient had an unremarkable travel history and no animal exposure, was a nonsmoker, and had no HIV risk factors. He worked for the power company cutting tree limbs and trees. On physical examination he was febrile to 38.3°C. The skin examination was notable for a tender, raised, erythematous papule (1 by 1 cm) on the bridge of the nose. A chest radiograph and subsequent chest CT scan were notable for a densely consolidated right middle lobe, a 3.5-cm subcarinal mass, and a small right hilar mass. Bronchoscopy was performed, and KOH, acid-fast, modified acid-fast, and Gram stains gave negative results. Examination of the lesion using a silver stain demonstrated a large, round budding yeast with a broad base connecting the mother cell to the daughter cell. (See Figure 12.)

1. What is the differential diagnosis for this patient's pulmonary disease?

2. Which organism is causing his illness? What are its epidemiology and culture characteristics?

3. This patient's lungs and skin were involved with this infection. Which other sites are commonly involved?

4. What in this patient's history might alert a physician to think of this organism?

5. Which organisms may be detected by a KOH examination? an acid-fast stain? a modified acid-fast stain?

DISCUSSION

1. The patient has a hilar mass and a densely consolidated right middle lobe. The differential diagnosis is the same as that discussed in case 40.

2. The agent of this individual's illness is *Blastomyces dermatitidis*. *B. dermatitidis* is a fairly large, broad-based budding yeast at body temperature (37°C). It is a dimorphic fungus, so at room or ambient temperature it grows as a mold. It is the etiologic agent of North American blastomycosis and should not to be confused with *Paracoccidioides brasiliensis*, the agent of South American blastomycosis. *B. dermatitidis* is endemic in much of the southeastern United States. Other regions where it is endemic include areas within the Mississippi and Ohio River basins and parts of western New York state and bordering areas in Canada.

3. Other sites that are frequently infected are bone, joints, and the genitourinary tract. In fact, this patient later developed multiple bone lesions. He presented with pain in his shins, and a bone scan showed multiple lesions, especially in his long bones. An aspirate of the bone lesion subsequently grew *B. dermatitidis*. He also is at risk for infection of the prostate and epididymis, both common complications of this infection.

4. The patient's symptoms are quite nonspecific. However, he failed to respond to three different regimens of antimicrobial therapy designed to treat common agents of community-acquired pneumonia such as *Mycoplasma pneumoniae* and *Streptococcus pneumoniae* and agents of bronchitis such as *Haemophilus influenzae* and *Moraxella catarrhalis*. The weight loss, low-grade fevers, and indolent clinical course are all suggestive of *Mycobacterium tuberculosis* infection. However, tuberculosis usually presents with upper lobe involvement, and a negative PPD skin test with positive skin test controls also argues against this infection. Patients with an indolent disease course and a nonproductive cough over extended periods frequently have pulmonary mycoses. The finding of the skin lesion on the face, a frequent occurrence in blastomycosis, further supports this diagnosis. The patient's occupation probably increased his risk for this infection. The organism can be recovered from decomposing wood. He probably was infected by inhaling spores while cutting down dead trees or branches. His skin infection was secondary to his primary pulmonary process.

5. On the basis of this patient's clinical presentation, a wide variety of microorganisms would be included in the differential diagnosis. Different techniques are required to best demonstrate the different organisms which would be considered. An acid-fast stain was done to detect mycobacteria.

Despite the negative skin test and atypical chest radiograph for tuberculosis, *M. tuberculosis* must still be considered as well as other mycobacteria. The modified acid-fast stain would be used to try to identify *Nocardia* spp., which could cause infections with a case presentation similar to this patient's. Finally, KOH is a commonly used technique to demonstrate fungi in clinical specimens. Fungi are fairly refractory to the activity of KOH, while human tissues are dissolved, clearing the specimen and making the microscopic demonstration of the fungi much easier. Other special stains (such as methenamine-silver or Calcofluor white) may demonstrate the presence of fungal elements in histologic specimens.

REFERENCES

Klein, B. S., J. M. Vergeront, A. F. DiSalvo, L. Kaufman, and J. P. Davis. 1987. Two outbreaks of blastomycosis along rivers in Wisconsin. Isolation of *Blastomyces dermatitidis* from riverbank soil and evidence of its transmission along waterways. *Am. Rev. Respir. Dis.* **136:**1333–1338.

Witorsch, P., and J. P. Utz. 1968. North American blastomycosis: a study of 40 patients. *Medicine* **47:**169–200.

This 52-year-old man was in his usual state of good health until approximately 1 year prior to hospital admission. At that time he noted that his right knee "tightened up" after he was working on his knees tending his nursery. Nine months prior to admission he consulted an orthopedic surgeon, and seven months prior to admission he underwent arthroscopy of his right knee. For a 6-week period following this procedure his knee improved, but then the tightness returned with swelling. The patient underwent physical therapy to help him extend the leg. His knee did not improve, and he sought further evaluation.

Physical examination was notable for a right knee effusion with warmth and mild tenderness. On range-of-motion testing, his knee extension was limited.

1. This patient has chronic arthritis with an infectious cause. What is the differential diagnosis of infectious causes of chronic arthritis?

2. Culture of arthrocentesis fluid was positive for a dimorphic fungus. When cultured at room temperature, the fungus grows as a darkly pigmented mold with slender hyphae. On growth at 37°C, the hyphae convert to round or spherical budding yeast cells. Although they were not noted on direct examination of fluid from this patient, cigar-shaped cells are occasionally found in infected tissue. What was the cause of this patient's infection?

3. Where in nature is this organism found? What in the patient's history is a clue to the cause of this infection?

4. What is the most common clinical presentation of infection with this organism? What are some of the less common ways in which infection with this agent may present?

DISCUSSION

1. The infectious causes of chronic arthritis include agents that grow slowly and evoke a granulomatous response from the host. These include mycobacterial infections with *Mycobacterium tuberculosis* and atypical mycobacteria, *Nocardia asteroides, Brucella* spp., and *Ureaplasma urealyticum* and fungal infections with agents such as *Sporothrix schenckii, Blastomyces dermatitidis, Coccidioides immitis,* and other fungi. Bacteria such as *Staphylococcus aureus, Neisseria gonorrhoeae,* and streptococci cause an acute suppurative arthritis, not a chronic arthritis.

2. *S. schenckii* was the fungus isolated from this patient.

3. *S. schenckii* is found in soil and plants. One common mechanism of infection is via inoculation by a thorn (e.g., from a rose during gardening) resulting in cutaneous disease. In this case, the patient, who worked on his knees tending a nursery, may have become infected by direct contact of his knee with plants and soil.

4. The most common type of infection is cutaneous sporotrichosis. A skin lesion occurs at the site of inoculation, and the infection may progress with the formation of new cutaneous lesions via lymphangitic spread. The diagnosis can be established by culture and histologic examination of a skin biopsy. Less commonly (as in this case), infection involves a bone or joint. Pulmonary sporotrichosis, ocular sporotrichosis, and disseminated sporotrichosis are extremely rare manifestations of infection with this organism.

REFERENCES

Urabe, H., and S. Honbo. 1986. Sporotrichosis. *Int. J. Dermatol.* **25**:255.
Wilson, D. E., J. J. Mann, J. E. Bennett, and J. P. Utz. 1967. Clinical features of extracutaneous sporotrichosis. *Medicine* **46**:265–279.

This 68-year-old North Carolina man with diabetes mellitus was admitted to the hospital for evaluation of a persistent right lower lobe infiltrate and treatment of diabetic ketoacidosis. Three weeks prior to admission, he presented to an outside physician for evaluation of fever, chills, weight loss, and anorexia. A chest radiograph demonstrated a right lower lobe infiltrate. He was treated with oral amoxicillin, but his condition worsened. His PPD test was negative, and three sputum specimens were negative for acid-fast bacilli on smear. Sputum specimens were sent for fungal culture. The patient works in a cotton mill in the so-called "opening room," where he opens bundles of cotton received from the southwestern United States.

He was initially treated for diabetic ketoacidosis. Cultures of sputum and blood grew a whitish mold which on microscopic examination had alternating, barrel-shaped arthroconidia. (See Figure 13.) Examination and culture of cerebrospinal fluid were unremarkable.

1. What is the fungus causing this man's illness? Which other microorganisms should be in this patient's differential diagnosis?

2. What is the geographic distribution of this fungus in the United States? What is its natural habitat?

3. If this man did not live in or travel to an area endemic for this fungus, how might he have become infected with this organism?

4. Which characteristic of this agent makes it highly infectious? How does the organism differ when grown in the environment and in a human host?

DISCUSSION

1. This patient has coccidioidomycosis caused by the dimorphic fungus *Coccidioides immitis*. This patient had a standard work-up for *Mycobacterium tuberculosis* which would have a similar clinical presentation except that lesions are more typically found in the upper lobes in patients with tuberculosis. Other organisms should be considered, such as *Francisella* spp., *Chlamydia psittaci*, *Brucella* spp., *Coxiella burnetii*, and *Legionella pneumophila*. A history of appropriate exposure or travel history would be required for several of these agents. The extended clinical course makes many of these agents less likely since the course of infection with many of them tends to be more acute. Other fungal agents such as *Histoplasma capsulatum* and *Blastomyces dermatitidis* would be more likely than *C. immitis* in North Carolina and would cause a clinical course similar to the one described here.

2. This organism is endemic in the southwestern United States and northern Mexico. Its natural habitat is soil. It grows particularly well in semiarid to arid regions which have alkaline soil, an ecosystem found in the Southwest. It is estimated to infect approximately 100,000 individuals annually in the United States. Most individuals will either be infected asymptomatically or have a flulike illness ("valley fever") that resolves spontaneously. Only a small percentage (<5%) will go on to have more extensive and prolonged pulmonary disease. Fewer still (<0.1%) will have disseminated disease, as was seen in this patient. Generally speaking, patients with diabetes tend to get more serious infections than do other individuals.

3. It is speculated that the patient inhaled arthroconidia of *C. immitis* which were present in the cotton he was handling. Cotton has been shown to be a vehicle for this infection in regions remote from the endemic area. This is an extraordinarily unusual means of acquiring infection compared with acquiring it in the region of endemicity.

4. The ability of this organism to produce easily aerosolized arthroconidia is the reason for its highly infectious nature. Arthroconidia are formed by the fragmentation of hyphae during sporulation. Mycelial growth is seen at ambient temperature, and it is the hyphal fragmentation into arthroconidia at this temperature which makes this organism so dangerous. When growing in a human host, the organism produces a yeastlike phase which is described as an endosporulating spherule. It should be emphasized that the in vivo phase of *C. immitis* is yeastlike and is not infectious to others. Because of the highly infectious nature of the mycelial phase of this organism, however, plates containing fluffy, white growth without other distinguishing features should be considered possible *C. immitis*

isolates. These plates should be sealed and handled only in laminar-flow safety cabinets.

REFERENCES

Knoper, S. R., and J. N. Galgiani. 1988. Systemic fungal infections: diagnosis and treatment. I. Coccidiomycosis. *Infect. Dis. Clin. N. Am.* **2:**861–875.

Labadie, E. L., and R. H. Hamilton. 1986. Survival improvement in coccidioidal meningitis by high-dose intrathecal amphotericin B. *Arch. Intern. Med.* **146:**2013–2018.

Table 2. Medically important fungi

Molds
  Aspergillus sp.
  Zygomycetes
    Mucor sp.
    Rhizopus sp.
    Rhizomucor sp.
    Cunninghamella sp.
  Dermatophytes
    Trichophyton sp.
    Microsporum sp.
    Epidermophyton sp.
  Fusarium sp.
  Pseudallescheria boydii

Yeasts
  Candida species
    Candida albicans
    Candida sp.
  Torulopsis glabrata
  Cryptococcus neoformans
  Trichosporon beigelii
  Malassezia furfur

Dimorphic fungi
  Blastomyces dermatitidis
  Coccidioides immitis
  Histoplasma capsulatum
  Paracoccidioides brasiliensis
  Sporothrix schenckii

This 29-year-old male was admitted for evaluation of a 2-week history of nonproductive cough, fever, and shortness of breath on minimal exertion. The patient has been actively homosexual since age 15 and has reportedly had more than 100 sexual partners. He sought medical attention from an outside physician and was given oral amoxicillin. His cough persisted, and he developed a rash while taking the amoxicillin. He went to a dermatologist, who took a chest radiograph, which was abnormal, demonstrating bilateral pulmonary infiltrates with both interstitial and alveolar markings. The patient was referred to the hospital emergency room. On examination, the patient was febrile to 38.3°C and had a respiratory rate of 24/min. Laboratory studies were remarkable for an arterial blood gas (obtained while the patient was breathing room air) with a pO$_2$ of 56 mmHg. The patient was treated with intravenous trimethoprim-sulfamethoxazole and underwent bronchoscopy with bronchoalveolar lavage.

1. This patient's sexual history placed him at high risk for infection with which virus?

2. What is the differential diagnosis of pulmonary infiltrates in patients who are infected with this virus?

3. A silver-stained preparation of bronchoalveolar lavage fluid demonstrated cysts. (See Figure 14.) What is the etiology of this individual's pulmonary infection? What are the diagnostic steps usually taken to detect this organism in the lungs?

4. What is the epidemiology of infection with the organism causing his pulmonary process? Does it cause clinically apparent infections in immunologically intact individuals? How does the virus identified in question 1 predispose this individual to his pulmonary infection?

5. Which pathologic event led to the low pO$_2$ in this patient?

6. How is infection with this organism treated? In patients at increased risk of infection, how is it prevented?

DISCUSSION

1. Patients who have multiple sexual partners, regardless of their sexual orientation, are at increased risk for infection with human immunodeficiency virus (HIV). Other viruses which can be transmitted sexually in patients with multiple sexual partners include herpes simplex virus, hepatitis B virus, human papillomavirus, and cytomegalovirus.

2. Patients who are infected with HIV are at increased risk of pneumonia caused by routine bacteria (such as *Streptococcus pneumoniae* and *Haemophilus influenzae*), mycobacteria (such as *Mycobacterium tuberculosis*), fungi (especially *Cryptococcus neoformans*), and parasites (in particular *Pneumocystis carinii*). Noninfectious causes of pulmonary infiltrates in HIV-positive patients include Kaposi's sarcoma and lymphoma.

3. This patient has *P. carinii* pneumonia (PCP) secondary to advanced-stage HIV disease. A variety of approaches to the diagnosis of this infection can be taken. The least invasive and least expensive diagnostic approach is to examine an induced sputum sample for the presence of the typical *P. carinii* cysts. Conventional sputum examination gives a low yield since sputum production is usually scanty in this disease. Sputum is induced by aerosolization of 3% saline into the airways, causing irritation which results in coughing and expectoration of lower respiratory tract secretions. Because the parasite burden is so high in HIV-infected patients, this technique has a sensitivity of 60 to 80%. Sputum induction for detection of *P. carinii* cysts in other immunocompromised patient populations has not been widely used and is believed to be of low yield. If induced sputum yields negative results in HIV-infected individuals, bronchoscopic examination is the next step. Bronchoalveolar lavage, as was used in this case, has a higher diagnostic yield than other types of bronchoscopic examinations and induced sputum. In bronchoalveolar lavage, large volumes of normal saline (100 to 200 ml) are introduced into a single lobe of the lung. This material lavages the bronchi and alveoli and is recovered by aspiration through the bronchoscope. This technique has a diagnostic yield of 90 to 95% for PCP. In selected patients with a negative bronchoalveolar lavage examination, open-lung biopsies may be performed. This technique is considered definitive for detection of PCP. Biopsies are useful for detecting other agents of pneumonia as well, if appropriate cultures and stains are used.

4. Serologic surveys suggest that *P. carinii* exposure or infection occurs early in childhood. Whether the organism remains dormant within the respiratory tract throughout life or actually is introduced at the time of infection

by inhalation is not entirely clear. What is clear is that immunologically intact individuals do not clinically manifest respiratory infections due to this organism. Cell-mediated immunity (CMI) appears to be protective, and only when disruptions in CMI occur are patients at increased risk for PCP. Because HIV disrupts CMI by causing a decline in the number of T-helper cells, PCP is a common infection in this patient population. In fact, AIDS was first recognized when an unusual cluster of PCP cases were seen in homosexual men in southern California. Approximately 60% of patients have PCP as their presenting sign of AIDS. Other patients at risk for PCP pneumonia include transplant recipients and patients with hematologic malignancies.

5. Oxygen exchange is extremely poor in the lungs of PCP patients because the organism causes the formation of a proteinaceous exudate in the alveoli. Proper oxygen exchange cannot occur in these fluid-filled spaces.

6. First-line therapy for this infection consists of intravenous trimethoprim-sulfamethoxazole. It has recently been recognized that short-course corticosteroid therapy in patients with significantly impaired oxygenation (such as this patient), in addition to antibiotics, is of benefit. Since many HIV-infected individuals experience side effects during therapy with sulfonamides, other antibiotics are frequently used. These include pentamadine, trimethoprim-dapsone, and several other experimental compounds. Prophylaxis against this infection, which is indicated in HIV-positive patients with fewer than 200 CD4-positive cells/mm^3, consists of oral trimethoprim-sulfamethoxazole daily or three times per week or nebulized pentamadine monthly.

REFERENCES

Bigby, T. D., D. Margolskee, J. L. Curtis, P. F. Michael, D. Sheppard, W. K. Hadley, and P. C. Hopewell. 1986. The usefulness of induced sputum in the diagnosis of *Pneumocystis carinii* pneumonia in patients with the acquired immunodeficiency syndrome. *Am. Rev. Respir. Dis.* **133:**515–518.

Bozzette, S. A., F. R. Sattler, J. Chiu, A. W. Wu, D. Gluckstein, C. Kemper, A. Bartok, J. Niosi, I. Abramson, J. Coffman, C. Hughlett, R. Loya, B. Cassens, B. Akil, T.-C. Meng, C. T. Boylen, D. Nielsen, D. D. Richman, J. G. Tilles, J. Leedom, J. A. McCutchan, and the California Collaborative Treatment Group. 1990. A controlled trial of early adjunctive treatment with corticosteroids for *Pneumocystis carinii* pneumonia in the acquired immunodeficiency syndrome. *N. Engl. J. Med.* **323:**1451–1457.

This 12-year-old boy was brought in by his mother for evaluation. The patient had been having crampy abdominal pain and some diarrhea for the preceding 1 to 2 weeks. On the afternoon of his evaluation, the patient thought that he had had an "accident" in his pants. When he looked in his underpants, he saw "something move" that his mother "captured." She told his pediatrician that she thought she had recovered "an earthworm." (See Figure 15.) He had no fever, cough, or blood-tinged sputum. His travel history was unremarkable. Physical examination was unremarkable as well, and no other worms or larvae were seen on anal examination.

1. Which human parasites are nematodes?

2. Which parasite was probably found in this patient?

3. How does one acquire infections with this parasite?

4. Describe the life cycle of this parasite.

5. Which organs can it invade? What symptoms can it cause?

DISCUSSION

1. The medically important intestinal nematodes include the etiologic agents of hookworm infection (*Necator americanus* and *Ancylostoma duodenale*), the pinworm (*Enterobius vermicularis*), the whipworm (*Trichuris trichiura*), the roundworm (*Ascaris lumbricoides*), and *Strongyloides stercoralis*. *Trichinella spiralis*, the etiologic agent of trichinosis, is not found in the feces.

2. The worm, which was submitted to the parasitology laboratory, was identified as *Ascaris lumbricoides*, the human roundworm. This nematode, when mature, may measure up to 35 cm in length. Diagnosis of ascariasis is most commonly made by identifying eggs in a fecal specimen. Females may contain millions of eggs and may lay as many as 200,000 eggs per day. Fertilized eggs are oval and up to 75 µm long; unfertilized eggs are elongated and up to 90 µm long.

3. Humans become infected by ingesting eggs after the eggs have matured in the soil. Thus the route of infection is fecal-oral. This infection is very common (there are approximately one billion infected people worldwide). Fecal contamination of soil and the use of human feces as fertilizer (as in many developing countries) help to explain the increased prevalence in regions of the world where these practices are common. Many other mammals are hosts to various ascarids, and humans can become an accidental host to these as well. This phenomenon is referred to as zoonotic infection, i.e., the acquisition by humans of an infectious agent which is found primarily in animals. The dog roundworm, *Toxocara canis*, and the cat roundworm, *Toxocara cati*, cause a syndrome referred to as visceral larva migrans.

4. Fertilized eggs are excreted by humans in feces. After 5 to 10 days in soil, the embryonated eggs are infectious. Once these infective eggs are swallowed, they hatch in the stomach and the small intestine. The larvae penetrate the intestinal wall and migrate via the portal circulation to the liver and then to the right heart, the pulmonary vessels, and the lungs. The larvae develop in the lungs and migrate up the bronchi and trachea and are swallowed. They mature in the intestines to the mature male and female and live in the lumen of the intestine, where females then lay eggs and begin the cycle again.

5. In addition to causing the common asymptomatic infections, *Ascaris* infection can affect the gastrointestinal tract. The clinical spectrum ranges from intermittent cramps to malnutrition to intestinal or biliary obstruction that may result in death. Worms may lodge in the appendix. The liver and

pancreas may be involved. As with many other parasitic infections that migrate through various tissues, eosinophilia may occur in patients with ascariasis. Pulmonary symptoms may occur during the migration of the larvae through the lungs and may simulate asthma or pneumonia. Worms may also migrate into other locations (such as the lacrimal duct or fallopian tubes), but this is uncommon.

REFERENCES

Blumenthal, D. S., and M. G. Schultz. 1974. Incidence of intestinal obstruction in children infected with *Ascaris lumbricoides*. *Am. J. Trop. Med. Hyg.* **24:**801–805.
Stephenson, L. S. 1980. The contribution of *Ascaris lumbricoides* to malnutrition in children. *Parasitology* **81:**221–233.

This 31-year-old man was referred for evaluation of diarrhea. Two months prior to admission the patient noted the onset of vague, crampy abdominal pain. At that time he developed profuse, watery diarrhea (8 to 10 stools per day). The diarrhea was often explosive. His work-up included negative stool cultures for bacterial pathogens, a normal flexible sigmoidoscope examination, and normal thyroid function tests. A stool specimen was sent for ova and parasites examination and demonstrated pear-shaped trophozoites 12 to 15 μm long with two bilateral nuclei (see Figure 16) and ovoid cysts 8 to 12 μm long with two or four nuclei.

1. Which parasite was found in the stool specimen? Other than detection in stool, which method can be used to diagnose this infection?

2. How is this parasite transmitted?

3. How can infection with this organism be prevented?

4. Other than chronic diarrhea (as in this patient), which symptoms can this parasite cause?

DISCUSSION

1. The trophozoites and cysts were those of the flagellate protozoan *Giardia lamblia*. The stool specimen demonstrated the free-living trophozoite, which contains four pairs of flagella and two nuclei, and cysts, which have two nuclei when immature and four when mature. In cases in which *G. lamblia* infection is suspected but not detected in daily stool specimens obtained over a 3-day period, the diagnosis is often established by examining duodenal contents by a method known as the string test. In this test the patient swallows a capsule containing a nylon string. The capsule is retrieved after 3 to 4 h, during which time it has entered the duodenum, the primary site of *Giardia* infection. The bile-stained string portion is examined for the presence of *Giardia* trophozoites. Aspiration of duodenal contents can also be performed to obtain diagnostic material.

2. Ingestion of cysts is required for the initiation of infection. Both animals and humans can serve as a source of *Giardia* cysts. In children in day-care settings, the cysts are most often transmitted directly from person to person. Since the infection is spread via the fecal-oral route, people who engage in direct anal-oral contact are also at increased risk of infection. In other persons, infection is often due to contaminated water or food. Hikers and campers can acquire infection from drinking water from mountain streams. One must always keep in mind that when drinking from a stream, there may always be at least one animal upstream contaminating the water. Various other mammals, especially beavers, have been implicated as reservoir hosts for *Giardia* spp.; therefore giardiasis may also be a zoonosis. Municipal water supplies have also been linked to outbreaks of disease. Because *Giardia* spp. are relatively resistant to chlorine, these outbreaks have occurred in cities that treat their potable water with chlorine rather than by filtration.

3. Individuals can prevent direct person-to-person (fecal-oral) spread by good hygiene practices (hand-washing). Communities must treat their water supplies appropriately to ensure that they are free of *Giardia* spp. People who travel in areas in which the water supply is suspect (e.g., mountain streams) should either boil the water or treat it with iodine. Likewise, food that has been washed in potentially contaminated water should be cooked prior to consumption.

4. In addition to chronic diarrhea, this parasite can produce an asymptomatic infection in which cysts are excreted in the stools. Another clinical picture that can result is that of acute diarrhea. Some patients with chronic diarrhea will have malabsorption as well. This is of particular concern in infants and young children in whom the malabsorptive syndrome is first

thought to be a milk allergy or lactose intolerance. The water supply for the child often is a well that is found to be fecally contaminated.

REFERENCES

Nash, T. E., D. A. Herrington, G. A. Losonsky, and M. M. Levine. 1987. Experimental human infections with *Giardia lamblia. J. Infect. Dis.* **156:**974–984.

Rosenthal, P., and W. M. Liebman. 1980. Comparative study of stool exams, aspiration, and pediatric Entero-Test for giardiasis in children. *J. Pediatr.* **96:**278–279.

This 28-year-old woman, known to be seropositive for HIV-1, presented with a complaint of diarrhea for more than 2 months. The diarrhea was described as watery, brown, and nonbloody and occurred every 5 min for up to 2 h after meals. She noted an 8-kg weight loss over this time, and the diarrhea did not respond to treatment with Kaopectate, Imodium, or Pepto-Bismol.

Physical examination was notable for orthostatic hypotension that was thought to be consistent with dehydration. A stool culture was negative for bacterial enteric pathogens. Examination of the stool for white blood cells gave negative results. The stool sample was also negative for *Clostridium difficile* toxin. A subsequent examination of the stool sample demonstrated acid-fast oocysts.

1. Which parasite was found in the patient's stool specimen?

2. How is infection with this organism transmitted?

3. Does infection occur among people with a normal immune system?

4. Patients such as this one can have such severe diarrhea that they become dehydrated. Some patients can have several liters of diarrhea per day. How can this occur?

5. There is currently no effective cure for this infection. AIDS patients are given fluid replacement and antidiarrheal medication which is helpful in some cases. How can the spread of infection from patient to patient be prevented in the hospital?

DISCUSSION

1. The protozoan *Cryptosporidum* spp. was the cause of this patient's diarrhea. Infection with this parasite can be diagnosed by staining stool specimens with a modified acid-fast stain that demonstrates oocysts. *Isospora* spp. and cyanobacter (blue-green algae), both known to cause diarrheal disease, are also acid fast. They are seen much less frequently as agents of diarrheal disease in HIV-infected individuals.

2. *Cryptosporidium* spp. are transmitted via the fecal-oral route. Many animal species can be infected with this parasite, and animal-to-human transmission, as well as human-to-human transmission (e.g., in day-care centers), occurs. Unfortunately, routine chlorination of water does not kill the oocyst, and contaminated water can be a source of infection. Following the ingestion of an oocyst, sporozoites within the oocysts excyst. A cycle of asexual reproduction followed by sexual reproduction ultimately results in the formation of oocysts, which are passed in the feces.

3. Although the diarrhea is most commonly seen in patients with AIDS, immunologically normal persons can be infected as well. This parasite has been shown to cause self-limited diarrheal disease in children attending day-care centers, and it also has been implicated as a cause of traveler's diarrhea.

4. The severe diarrhea that can occur in patients with cryptosporidiosis is a secretory diarrhea. Secretory diarrhea is characterized by severe fluid loss (up to several liters per day) and an absence of white blood cells in the feces. The best-studied secretory diarrhea is that in cholera, in which massive diarrhea due to activation of adenylate cyclase by cholera toxin may lead to dehydration and, if untreated, death. Although *Cryptosporidium* spp. produce typical pathologic lesions in the small intestine (referred to as pedestal formation), no toxin has been found. The biochemical events that lead to this debilitating secretory diarrhea are unknown.

5. Prevention of the spread of cryptosporidiosis (as with other diarrheal diseases) within a health care setting is dependent upon, first and foremost, good hygiene practices (hand-washing).

REFERENCES

Soave, R., and D. Armstrong. 1986. *Cryptosporidium* and cryptosporidiosis. *Rev. Infect. Dis.* **8**:1012–1023.
Wolfson, J. S., J. M. Richter, M. A. Waldron, D. J. Weber, D. M. McCarthy, and C. C. Hopkins. 1985. Cryptosporidiosis in immunocompetent patients. *N. Engl. J. Med.* **312**:1278–1282.

The patient was a 22-year-old male with classic hemophilia (factor VIII deficiency) who is monitored at our hospital. He presented to an outside hospital for evaluation of nausea, vomiting, and increasing headache. A head CT scan at that time demonstrated ring-enhancing lesions in the right parietal lobe. The neurosurgical service performed a biopsy of the brain lesions. Bacterial, fungal, and viral cultures were all negative. Special stains of the biopsy specimen revealed cysts which varied greatly in size.

1. What is the likely etiology of this patient's infection?

2. Do you think this patient is immunocompetent? Explain your answer.

3. How should this patient be managed?

4. Would you expect this patient to have any pets? Explain your answer.

5. In France, the seroprevalence rate for this organism is extremely high. Why is this?

6. Why is it important for pregnant women to avoid infection with this organism? What measures would you advise a pregnant woman to take to avoid this infection?

DISCUSSION

1. This patient has a brain lesion as evidenced by his clinical presentation and the CT findings. The differential diagnosis in this patient would include infection with *Toxoplasma gondii*, *Cryptococcus neoformans*, mixed aerobic and anaerobic bacteria (brain abscess), *Nocardia* spp., and *Mycobacterium* spp. Brain tumors and primary central nervous system (CNS) lymphoma should also be considered. Because of the wide range of possibilities which require quite different treatment strategies, it was determined that a brain biopsy was necessary. The biopsy revealed the diagnosis of *T. gondii*. In many cases HIV-positive patients with multiple ring-enhancing lesions are treated empirically for toxoplasmosis and monitored rather than being subjected to a brain biopsy. This organism will form cysts of various sizes in the brain.

2. Specific factors in this case suggest that this patient is not immunocompetent. First, he is a hemophilic who received factor VIII prior to its pasteurization. This means that he is in a high-risk group for HIV infection. At our institution (which is a large hemophilia center), approximately 60% of the hemophilics (including this patient) are HIV positive. In immunocompetent individuals *T. gondii* infections are typically asymptomatic or extremely mild and self-limited. However, in immunodeficient patients, *T. gondii* infections can be quite severe. The most frequent, serious manifestation is *T. gondii* encephalitis, as was seen in this patient. It is estimated that 5 to 10% of patients with AIDS in the United States develop this infection.

3. Cell-mediated immunity (CMI) is necessary for resolution of *T. gondii* infection. Because patients with AIDS have profoundly depressed CMI, they often relapse once chemotherapeutic agents used to treat this infection are withdrawn. As a result, chemotherapy with pyrimethamine and sulfadiazine for serious *T. gondii* infection must be continued for life in these patients.

4 and 5. It would not be surprising to learn that this patient has a cat (as do millions of people in the United States) or has been exposed to cats in the past. Cats are the definitive host for *T. gondii*, and they excrete the oocyst of this organism in their feces. After a brief period in the environment, these oocysts become infectious and individuals can become infected by ingesting them. Alternatively, tissue cysts can be found in pork, lamb, and beef. The practice of eating rare or raw meat in France is believed to explain, at least in part, the comparatively high seropositivity rate in that country.

6. In addition to horizontal transmission from animals to humans, *T. gondii* can be transmitted vertically from a mother to her fetus. The infection is generally asymptomatic in the mother when it is contracted during pregnancy. Infection of the fetus is often devastating, causing fetal wastage or various birth defects including blindness, epilepsy, hydrocephalus, and mental retardation.

Women who are seropositive prior to conception are unlikely to transmit this organism to their fetuses, so it is incumbent on only seronegative women who become pregnant to take precautions to avoid *T. gondii* infection. These include thoroughly cooking meat and vegetables (which may be fecally contaminated), wearing gloves when working with soil, and disposing of cat litter daily before oocysts can sporulate and become infectious. As with all infectious diseases spread by the fecal-oral route, hand-washing after contact with soil, animals, and animal feces helps decrease the risk of transmission.

REFERENCES

Daffos, F., F. Forestier, M. Capella-Pavlovsky, P. Thulliez, C. Aufrant, D. Valenti, and W. Cox. 1988. Prenatal management of 746 pregnancies at risk of congenital toxoplasmosis. *N. Engl. J. Med.* **318:**271–275.

Wong, G., J. M. Gold, A. E. Brown, M. Lange, R. Fried, M. Grieco, D. Mildvan, J. Giron, M. L. Tapper, C. W. Lerner, and D. Armstrong. 1984. Central nervous system toxoplasmosis in homosexual men and parenteral drug abusers. *Ann. Intern. Med.* **100:**36–42.

This 21-year-old man, who emigrated from Mexico 3 years prior to admission, was in his usual state of good health until the day of admission, when he had a witnessed seizure and was taken via ambulance to an outside emergency room. Neurologic examination demonstrated no focal findings. A head CT scan was performed; it was remarkable for the presence of multiple small cystic and punctate calcified lesions in both cerebral hemispheres.

The patient was transferred to a university hospital, where a lumbar puncture was performed. The CSF was notable for 22 nucleated cells/mm^3 with a differential of 7% neutrophils, 88% lymphocytes, and 5% monocytes. The CSF glucose level was 63 mg/dl, and the CSF protein level was 36 mg/dl. A PPD skin test was negative with a positive tetanus toxoid control.

1. What is the differential diagnosis of this patient's intracranial process?

2. Serum and CSF were sent for serologic studies to the Centers for Disease Control, where the clinical diagnosis was confirmed serologically. What is the likely diagnosis?

3. Which parasite causes this infection?

4. How do people become infected with this parasite? What in this patient's history indicates that he is at increased risk for this infection?

5. Other than the central nervous system, which organs may be involved in infection with this parasite?

DISCUSSION

1 and 2. The presence of multiple intracranial lesions is consistent with a noninfectious process, such as cancer with metastases to the brain, as well as with several infectious processes. Multiple brain lesions would be consistent with central nervous system toxoplasmosis in an immuno-compromised host. This patient was found to be negative for antibody to HIV and had no apparent immunosuppression, so toxoplasmosis was ruled out. Although central nervous system tuberculosis occasionally pre-sents with tuberculomas in the brain, a PPD skin test was performed with negative results. Multiple brain abscesses are another possibility. None of these possibilities would adequately explain the radiologic findings. These are best explained by cerebral cysticercosis. Indeed, as part of this patient's evaluation, serologic studies were performed by the Centers for Disease Control, which confirmed the diagnosis of cysticercosis. Both serum and cerebrospinal fluid should be sent for serologic studies in the setting of suspected cerebral cysticercosis.

3. Infection with the embryonic form of the parasite *Taenia solium*, the pork tapeworm, causes cysticercosis. Infection with the beef tapeworm, *Taenia saginata*, does not cause cysticercosis.

4. Following the ingestion of contaminated undercooked pork, cysticercus larvae are liberated in the stomach. The adult tapeworm subsequently establishes itself in the human small intestine. *T. solium* eggs are excreted in the feces of carriers. Following the ingestion of food contaminated with *T. solium* eggs, gastric acid and pancreatic enzymes cause the release of oncospheres (motile larva) that penetrate the intestinal wall and are dis-seminated in the blood. This dissemination occurs only following inges-tion of the eggs and does not follow ingestion of cysts. Cysticercosis is common in Mexico and is a major cause of a new seizure disorder in adults in that country. *T. solium* is common in pigs in Mexico and other Latin American countries.

5. In addition to the presence of the adult worm in the small intestine, the larval stage (cysticercus) may be found in many sites in the body. Most commonly the larvae disseminate to the muscles, eyes, and brain. In the pig, they spread to the muscles as well. Once the muscle (if it is un-dercooked) is eaten by a human, the cycle can start again.

REFERENCE

Del Brutto, O. H., and J. Sotelo. 1988. Neurocysticercosis: an update. *Rev. Infect. Dis.* **10**:1075–1087.

CASE 50

This 35-year-old female was admitted to the hospital in transfer from the student health service. The patient had been in Zambia for the 8 months prior to admission. She was hospitalized there, 1 month prior to admission, with fever, malaise, and headaches and was treated empirically with chloroquine. The patient initially felt better, but was rehospitalized 2 weeks prior to admission. Laboratory studies performed in Zambia were consistent with the diagnosis of malaria. The patient's condition again improved with chloroquine therapy, and she returned to the United States 2 days prior to admission. She presented with renewed onset of fever, malaise, and headaches.

1. On the basis of the geographic distribution and clinical course, which *Plasmodium* species is likely to be the cause of infection? What other *Plasmodium* species are there, and what are their geographic distributions?

2. Give the most likely reason why the chloroquine did not cure this patient's malaria. How does her clinical course support your explanation?

3. Which laboratory test(s) would confirm the diagnosis of malaria?

4. Which *Plasmodium* species causes the most severe disease? Discuss a serious complication of infection with this parasite.

5. How is malaria transmitted? What control measures are available to prevent its transmission?

DISCUSSION

1. The most likely *Plasmodium* species to be found in Central Africa are *Plasmodium falciparum* and, to a much lesser extent, *P. ovale*. *P. falciparum* was detected in this patient. *P. falciparum* is also frequently found in southeast Asia and South America. Other species of malaria include *P. vivax*, which is found primarily in the Indian subcontinent, southeast Asia, and Central and South Africa, and *P. malariae*, which has a worldwide distribution in malaria-endemic areas.

2. The presence of chloroquine-resistant strains of *P. falciparum* in Africa is well recognized, and it is likely that this patient was infected with a chloroquine-resistant strain. Her clinical course was consistent with chloroquine-resistant organisms. Patients infected with resistant organisms may show clinical improvement on chloroquine therapy only to relapse some time (days to weeks) after the end of therapy. The failure of chloroquine therapy is further evidence that this patient has a *P. falciparum* infection, since this is the only *Plasmodium* species for which widespread chloroquine resistance has been reported, although chloroquine-resistant *P. vivax* has also been recently identified.

3. The diagnosis of malaria can be made by examination of a stained smear of peripheral blood. A thin smear is made on a microscope slide. It is optimally one cell thick and thus allows the examination of parasitized red blood cells in sufficient detail to allow determination of the *Plasmodium* species that is causing the infection. In a light infection in which only a small percentage of red blood cells are parasitized, the smear may be negative for the parasite. A thick smear, which is many cells thick, can detect a parasitemia that may be undetectable in the thin smear. The thick smear is not as useful in examining the fine details of the parasite that help to make the diagnosis to the species level. Parasitemia is highest during malarial paroxysm (the high fever and shaking chills characteristic of this disease).

4. The species of malaria which causes the most severe disease is *P. falciparum*. Two severe complications of *P. falciparum* are cerebral malaria and blackwater fever. Cerebral malaria is currently believed to be a metabolic encephalopathy. This encephalopathy is thought to be due to cerebral anoxia coupled with increased glucose utilization and lactate production by infected erythrocytes which bind to endothelium in the cerebral vasculature. Clinically, these patients have altered states of consciousness, confusion, hallucinations, seizures, motor abnormalities, and coma. Blackwater fever is characterized by hemoglobinuria secondary to massive hemolysis. The events that trigger this massive hemolysis are not

clear. However, it may represent a hypersensitivity reaction to drugs used to treat the infection. Hepatic, renal, adrenal, and pulmonary complications may also be seen with severe infection.

5. The disease has been shown to be spread in one of two ways. The most common way is via an insect vector, the female *Anopheles* mosquito. While feeding on a human host, the mosquito can ingest malaria parasites (gametocytes). These parasites develop in the insect host over approximately 2 weeks, until the infectious phase of the parasite (sporozoite) migrates to the salivary glands of the insects. At the next blood meal, the sporozoites are injected into the blood of a human host. These sporozoites invade the liver, where they develop into merozoites, which in turn can enter the bloodstream and infect red blood cells, resulting in the parasitemia of malaria. Another, less frequent, way in which malaria can be spread is via blood transfusions from an infected to a noninfected individual. Therefore, individuals who return from malaria-endemic regions should refrain from donating blood for 3 years.

Three different strategies have been attempted for malaria control. One of the time-honored methods for the prevention of infection is vector control. This can be accomplished in two ways. The first way is by using insecticides. Unfortunately, there are numerous examples of the insect vector becoming resistant to insecticides. The second way is by using protective clothing and insect repellent and by sleeping under mosquito netting. The other time-honored approach is chemoprophylaxis for the suppression of infection. Chloroquine is taken every 7 days for 2 weeks before entering an area in which malaria is endemic, throughout the stay, and for 6 weeks after returning from the region. Prophylaxis for individuals entering areas with chloroquine-resistant *P. falciparum* is much more complex. Up-to-date recommendations on prophylaxis for persons entering these areas can be obtained from the Centers for Disease Control.

Finally, serious attempts are under way to develop malaria vaccines. Progress in developing such a vaccine has been slow, in part because of the exceedingly complex life cycle of the parasite. Each stage of the parasite has different surface antigens, and determining which stage and which surface antigens to use to induce immunity has been difficult. It also has been recognized that stimulation of both humoral and cell-mediated immunity is important in developing protective immunity. Small trials of candidate vaccines, to date, have not been particularly successful.

REFERENCES

Gordon, D. M. 1990. Malaria vaccines. *Infect. Dis. Clin. N. Am.* **4:**299–313.

Warrell, D. A., M. E. Molyneux, and P. F. Beales (ed.). 1990. Severe and complicated malaria. World Health Organization Division of Control of Tropical Diseases. *Trans. R. Soc. Trop. Med. Hyg.* **84**(Suppl. 2):1–65.

Table 3. Medically important parasites

Protozoa
  Amoebae
    Acanthamoeba spp.
    Endolimax nana
    Entamoeba coli
    Entamoeba hartmanni
    Entamoeba histolytica
    Naegleria fowleri

  Flagellates
    Giardia lamblia
    Leishmania spp.
    Trichomonas vaginalis

  Coccidiae
    Cryptosporidium spp.
    Isospora belli
    Toxoplasma gondii

  Sporozoae
    Plasmodium falciparum
    Plasmodium malariae
    Plasmodium ovale
    Plasmodium vivax
    Pneumocystis carinii

Platyhelminthes
  Cestodes
    Taenia saginata
    Taenia solium
    Echinococcus spp.

  Trematodes
    Schistosoma haematobium
    Schistosoma japonicum
    Schistosoma mansonii
    Schistosoma sp.

Aschelminthes
  Nematodes
    Ancylostoma duodenale
    Ascaris lumbricoides
    Enterobius vermicularis
    Necator americanus
    Onchocerca volvulus
    Strongyloides stercoralis
    Trichuris trichiura
    Trichinella spiralis

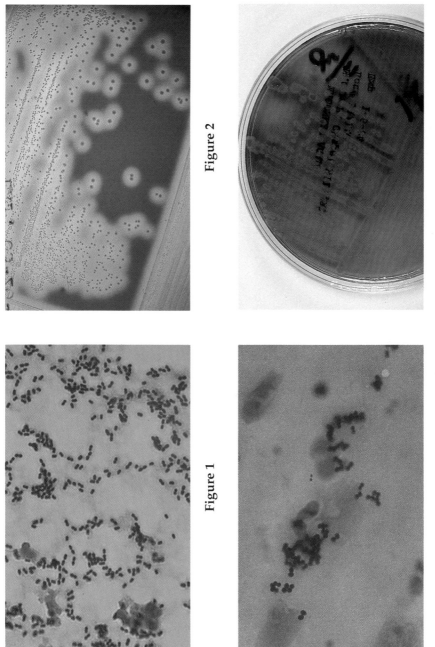

Figure 1

Figure 2

Figure 3

Figure 4

(Complete figure identification on page 259)

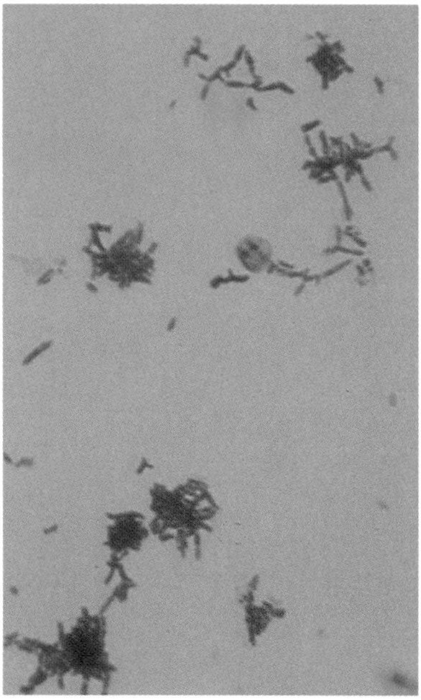

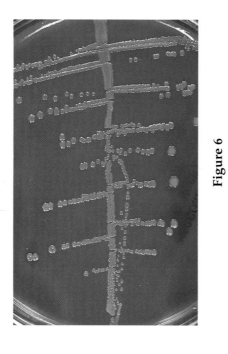

Figure 6

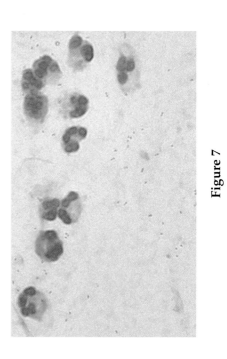

Figure 8

Figure 5

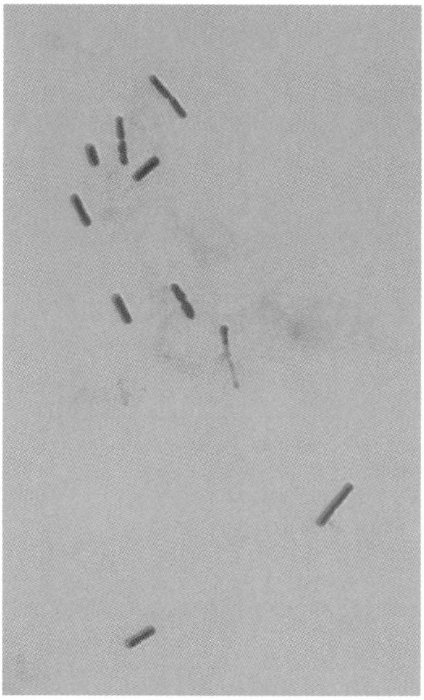

Figure 7

(Complete figure identification on page 259)

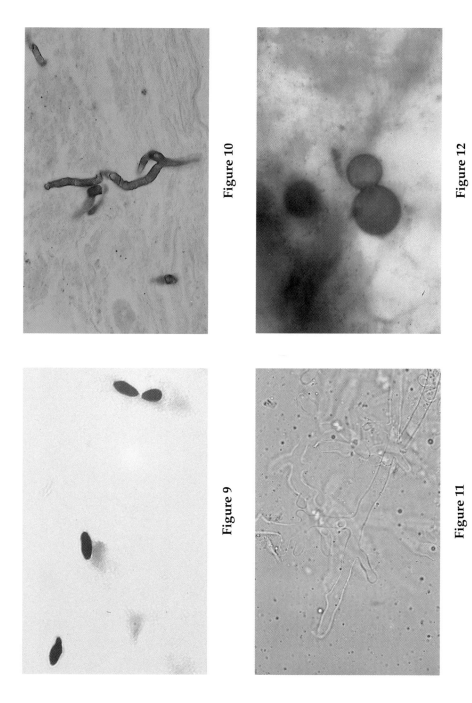

Figure 9

Figure 10

Figure 11

Figure 12

(Complete figure identification on page 259)

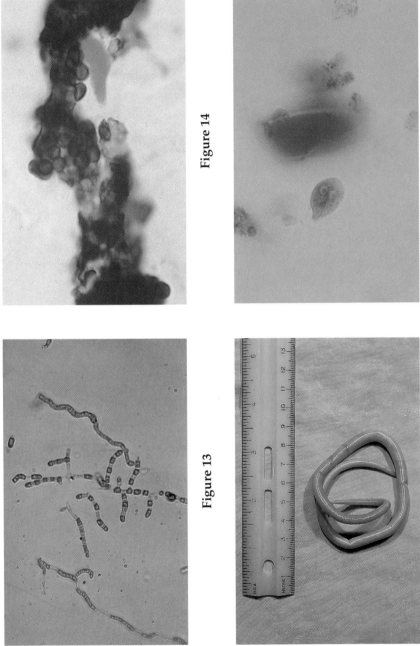

Figure 13

Figure 14

Figure 15

Figure 16

(Complete figure identification on page 259)

VIROLOGY

The discovery of the human immunodeficiency viruses (HIV-1 and HIV-2) as the cause of the acquired immunodeficiency syndrome (AIDS) has been one of the great medical achievements of the past decade. This accomplishment, along with an ever clearer understanding of the clinical importance of viral infection in the immuno-compromised host, has resulted in virology becoming a major focus of current medical inquiry. As certain viral infections are conquered by the use of vaccines (polio), new agents besides HIV are being recognized (parvovirus, hepatitis C, etc.), presenting new clinical and diagnostic challenges.

It should be emphasized that viral infections are very common and viruses cause a wide spectrum of disease ranging from the common cold to AIDS. Since antiviral agents are few and their activity is highly specific, public health strategies to control viral infections have focused on vaccine development and use.

In this section of the book, the commonly encountered diseases caused by viruses are emphasized. In addition, cases due to recently discovered viral agents are highlighted.

CASE 51

The patient was a 4-month-old female who was admitted to the hospital in March with severe respiratory distress. Five days prior to admission she had developed a cough and rhinitis. Two days later she began wheezing and was noted to have a fever. She was brought to the emergency room when she became lethargic.

One sibling was reported to be coughing, and her father had a "cold." On examination she was agitated and coughing. She had a fever of 38.9°C, tachycardia with a pulse of 220, tachypnea with respirations of 80/min, and a blood pressure of 90/58 mmHg. Her fontanelles were open, soft, and flat. Her throat was clear. She had subcostal retractions and nasal flaring. On auscultation of her lungs, there were rhonchi as well as inspiratory and expiratory wheezes.

A chest radiograph revealed interstitial infiltrates and hyperexpansion. Arterial blood gases on supplemental oxygen revealed a respiratory acidosis with relative hypoxemia. She was put in respiratory isolation in the pediatric intensive care unit and was subsequently intubated. Blood and nasopharyngeal cultures were obtained and sent to the bacteriology and virology laboratories. A rapid viral diagnostic test was positive, and specific antiviral therapy was begun. She was also given the bronchodilator aminophylline to treat her bronchospasm, which was resulting in her wheezing. She was extubated 5 days later and discharged home on day 8.

1. What is the differential diagnosis for this patient's croup, and which of the possible viral agents is the most likely etiology?

2. Of these possibilities, which one can be diagnosed by a specific rapid test for antigen?

3. Describe the pathophysiologic basis for her wheezing.

4. What specific therapy was given after the antigen test revealed the diagnosis?

5. What are the hospital's infection control issues related to this patient's diagnosis?

DISCUSSION

1. The differential diagnosis for this patient's pneumonia includes respiratory viruses such as parainfluenza virus types 1, 2, and 3, influenza A and B viruses, and respiratory syncytial virus (RSV). *Mycoplasma pneumoniae* or *Bordetella pertussis* could also have caused her illness. This patient was found to be infected with RSV, which causes severe infections in children less than 1 year old, whereas reinfections in older children and adults may result in minimal respiratory tract symptoms. RSV can also cause acute laryngotracheobronchitis (see case 53). The elderly may also develop severe RSV infections.

2. Rapid antigen detection tests are currently available for RSV, influenza A and B viruses, parainfluenza virus types 1 to 3, and adenovirus. RSV can be detected in nasopharyngeal washings or aspirates by either an enzyme immunoassay (EIA) or immunofluorescence. Many institutions are replacing immunofluorescence with EIA because EIA is easier to perform, is more rapid when multiple specimens must be tested, and has similar sensitivity and specificity. RSV isolation in cell culture takes 3 to 10 days. The advantage of culture is a higher degree of sensitivity than that of rapid procedures, and culture has the ability to detect a variety of viral agents. However, specimens for RSV culture must be quickly transported and cultured because this virus soon loses infectivity outside the host. Rapid viral antigen tests are valuable because of the length of time required to detect many viruses in culture. Prompt results are preferred so that the decision to use antiviral agents can be made as soon as possible.

3. Wheezing and stridorous cough develop in infants with RSV infection because the virus has a tropism for the bronchial epithelium. The diameter of an infant's bronchioles is small, and so edema and necrosis lead to collapse and obstruction which can result in air trapping distally. The lung parenchyma can be involved with or without the bronchiolitis. This patient apparently had involvement of both the bronchioles and the lung parenchyma.

4. Only one antiviral agent, ribavirin, is available for treatment of RSV in infants. It has been shown to decrease viral shedding and increase the patient's oxygenation. It must be delivered by aerosol since oral (p.o.) administration may result in hepatic or bone marrow toxicity.

5. Because RSV can cause nosocomial infections, patients should be put in respiratory isolation. If patients are not isolated and infection control practices (strict hand-washing, use of gloves and gowns, etc.) are not used, cross-infections can occur at a rate of 20 to 50%. Several patients with RSV can be "cohorted" (put in the same room), and their health care

providers can be similary cohorted. Nosocomial RSV infections are a hazard particularly for other hospitalized patients with congenital heart disease, lung disease, or immunodeficiency states who are at risk for life-threatening RSV infections.

REFERENCE

Smith, D. W., L. R. Frankel, L. H. Mathers, A. T. S. Tang, R. L. Ariagno, and C. G. Prober. 1991. A controlled trial of aerosolized ribavirin in infants receiving mechanical ventilation for severe respiratory syncytial virus infection. *N. Engl. J. Med.* 325:24–29.

The patient was a 14-year-old mentally retarded male with a history of a seizure disorder. He presented to his doctor in early January with a 5-day history of a fever, headache, nonproductive cough, nausea, vomiting, and lack of energy. He also had a loss of appetite, severe myalgias, and nasal congestion. The day he presented to his physician, he noted shortness of breath. On the same day, his mother became ill, having headache, fever, and myalgias. His physical examination was noteworthy for a temperature of 39°C and an increased respiratory rate of 35/min. He was dehydrated, and rales were heard at the base of his right lung. Laboratory data revealed normal electrolytes, creatinine, liver function tests, and complete blood count (CBC). His monospot test was negative. His creatine kinase level (CPK) was slightly elevated. Analysis of arterial blood gases showed mild hypoxemia and respiratory alkalosis. A chest radiograph revealed a right lower lobe infiltrate. An induced sputum sample was obtained and sent for routine bacterial culture and viral culture. The sputum Gram stain was unremarkable.

He was admitted and given supplemental oxygen and intravenous hydration. Oral erythromycin therapy was begun pending culture results. He was also given antipyretics. Over the next 4 days, steady improvement was noted. On the fifth hospital day, a viral culture result revealed the diagnosis.

1. What is the differential diagnosis? What is the most likely etiology? Describe the functions of the two known virulence factors of this virus.

2. What is the least appropriate antipyretic to use in order to manage his fever? Explain your answer.

3. What strategies are available to prevent infection with this virus? Why are changes made in one of these preventative strategies each year?

4. His father has emphysema. How should he be managed?

DISCUSSION

1. The differential diagnosis of viral respiratory diseases in adolescents and adults includes the following: influenza virus, parainfluenza virus, respiratory syncytial virus, rhinovirus, adenovirus, measles virus, coronaviruses, coxsackievirus, and echoviruses, as well as varicella-zoster virus, cytomegalovirus (immunocompromised hosts), and herpes simplex virus (special circumstances).

    This patient was not immunocompromised, and he developed an illness during the winter. Systemic symptoms were prominent, and he had evidence of lower respiratory tract involvement (pneumonia). His mother developed a similar illness. The most likely diagnosis is influenza, with parainfluenza a second possibility.

    Influenza virus is one of the best-understood viruses in terms of pathogenesis. It is an RNA virus which has a segmented genome and belongs to the myxovirus group. Two virulence factors are recognized for this virus, hemagglutinin and neuraminidase. Hemagglutinin binds the virus to epithelial cells in the respiratory tract. The role of neuraminidase is less clear. It may help attach the virus by degrading mucins in the respiratory tract, thus allowing access of the hemagglutinin to the epithelial cell surface. It has also been suggested that this enzyme may play a role in the release of the virus from the infected cell.

2. Aspirin should never be used in children or young adults with viral illnesses such as influenza or varicella. There is an association of aspirin usage with the development of Reye's syndrome. This syndrome is often fatal and includes severe hepatic and central nervous system complications.

    Acetaminophen is the appropriate antipyretic to use in this case.

3. There are two basic strategies for preventing influenza. First, annual vaccinations can prevent the majority of infections. Vaccines are made each year and include specific influenza A and B virus strains predicted to cause major illness. The need for yearly changes in the vaccine is due to the distinctive ability of this virus, especially influenza A, to change over time.

    Influenza virus can undergo alterations in the antigenicity of its two major surface antigens, hemagglutinin and neuraminidase. Relatively minor changes in surface antigens which occur frequently are referred to as antigenic drift. Antigenic drift is believed to be due to point mutation(s) in the RNA genome. It may lead to a selective advantage of the antigenically modified virus over the parent strain. Antibodies in patients exposed to the parent virus may be less protective against the mutated strain, allowing for its greater transmission. Antigenic shift is defined as major changes in the antigenic structure of hemagglutinin or neuraminidase or both. Antigenic shift occurs as result of genetic reassortment, in which genomic RNA segments are exchanged between viruses, leading to major changes in the antigenic structure of the virus. It results in an antigenically new virus. Populations may have no immunity to the new virus, and influenza epidemics may occur as a result of these viral changes. Fortunately, antigenic shift occurs infrequently, historically at 10- to 20-year intervals.

Because the virus can undergo both major and minor antigenic variation, vaccines are produced each year based on the prevalent strains of the previous year to ensure induction of the best possible immunity in at-risk populations. Yearly vaccination is recommended for individuals with chronic respiratory and cardiac disease, for those with immunodeficiencies, the elderly, and health care providers.

Second, the use of the antiviral agent amantadine may prevent some infections with influenza A virus but not influenza B virus.

4. His father has preexisting respiratory compromise and is at high risk for developing severe illness if he acquires influenza.

He should receive annual influenza vaccinations. In this particular situation he should also receive amantadine. If influenza B virus was isolated from his son, amantadine would be ineffective in preventing infection.

REFERENCES

Douglas, R. G. 1989. Influenza in the 1990's—use of antiviral agents in prophylaxis and treatment. *J. Respir. Dis.* **10**(Suppl):s19–s68.
Hurwitz, E. S., M. J. Barrett, D. Bregman, W. J. Gunn, L. B. Schonberger, W. R. Fairweather, J. S. Drage, J. R. LaMontagne, R. A. Kaslow, D. B. Burlington, G. V. Quinnan, R. A. Parker, K. Phillips, P. Pinsky, D. Dayton, and W. R. Dowdle. 1985. Public health service study on Reye's syndrome and medications. *N. Engl. J. Med.* **313**:849–857.

The patient was a 1-year-old male who was brought to the clinic in January because he developed fever, chest congestion, rhinorrhea, and a "barking" cough 3 days previously. His appetite was fair. There was no sputum production, nausea, or vomiting.

His medical history was significant only for recurrent otitis media. On examination, his temperature was 38.4°C. He was in no acute distress and had audible obstructive upper airway sounds. His throat was erythematous. On lung examination, upper airway sounds were prominent and there was no wheezing or subcostal retractions. The clinical impression was that he had croup. Specimens were sent for viral cultures. He was managed with therapies for symptomatic relief including the use of a humidifier in the home. Ten days later a virus was identified from a nasopharyngeal specimen only after hemabsorption studies were done on the virus culture.

1. What is the differential diagnosis, including viral and nonviral etiologies?

2. What are hemabsorption studies? Which group of viruses is freqently detected by this technique? Which virus in this group is most likely to cause the above clinical syndrome?

3. Describe the spectrum of clinical illnesses which can be caused by the virus infecting this patient.

4. What is the epidemiology of this virus?

5. What treatment and/or vaccines are available for this virus?

DISCUSSION

1. This patient's clinical diagnosis was croup (acute laryngotracheobronchitis). The pathophysiology of croup is due to infection and inflammation
in the subglottic area. This leads to a stridorous cough. Organisms which
can cause croup or a crouplike illness include parainfluenza virus (PIV),
RSV, influenza virus, *Corynebacterium diphtheriae, Haemophilus influenzae,
Mycoplasma pneumoniae,* and *Bordetella pertussis.*

2. Hemabsorption studies can be used to detect myxoviruses growing in
tissue culture cells. Myxoviruses are a large group of enveloped RNA
viruses including both orthomyxoviruses (influenza virus) and paramyx-
oviruses (PIV-1 to PIV-4, mumps virus, measles virus, and RSV). The
myxoviruses except for RSV produce hemagglutinins on the surface of the
infected cell. In hemabsorption studies, erythrocytes (RBCs) are applied to
the tissue culture cells and they are examined for RBC adherence. If
hemagglutinins are expressed on the cell monolayer, the RBCs will adhere
to them and thus the specimen will be hemabsorption positive. Cells
infected with myxoviruses are generally hemabsorption positive before
they show cytopathic changes, so hemabsorption studies can speed the
detection of these viruses in culture. Since hemabsorption can be nonspecific, many laboratories use specific monoclonal antibodies to differentiate
the viruses by fluorescent antibody assays.

    This patient was infected with parainfluenza virus type 1 (PIV-1). PIV is
the virus most commonly associated with croup. There are four serotypes of
PIV, PIV-1 to PIV-4. Like influenza virus, PIV produces both hemagglutinins
and neuraminidase. Unlike influenza virus, PIV has a nonsegmented ge-
nome and the four types are antigenically stable. RSV can cause a similar
clinical syndrome to PIV.

3. Manifestations of parainfluenza virus infections are generally more severe
in infants and young children than in adults. Infection can result in severe
pneumonia, bronchitis, laryngitis, croup (laryngotracheobronchitis), or
just a mild upper respiratory tract infection. There are no extrapulmonary
manifestations.

    Immunity is only transient. Repeat infections, which are usually milder,
occur in older children and adults.

4. Parainfluenza is a disease seen primarily in children 4 months to 6 years of
age. Epidemic disease occurs in the fall with PIV-1 or PIV-2 predominantly
in alternate years. PIV-3 appears to be endemic throughout the year. Like
all enveloped respiratory viruses, PIV is spread most efficiently by aerosolization.

5. Unlike the situation for influenza virus, there are no available vaccines or specific antiviral agents for parainfluenza virus. The disease is generally self-limited and requires only supportive care.

REFERENCES

Glezen, W. P., F. A. Loda, and F. W. Denny. 1984. Parainfluenza viruses, p. 441–454. *In* A. S. Evans (ed.), *Viral Infections of Humans: Epidemiology and Control.* Plenum Press, New York.

Hall, C. B. 1990. Acute laryngotracheitis (croup), p. 499–505. *In* G. L. Mandell, R. G. Douglas, Jr., and J. E. Bennett (ed.), *Principles and Practice of Infectious Disease,* 3rd ed. Churchill Livingstone, Inc., New York.

The patient was a 20-year-old female who presented to the emergency room with a 4-day history of fever, chills, and myalgia. Two days prior to this she noted painful genital lesions. On the day of admission she developed headache, photophobia, and a stiff neck. Previously, she had been in good health. She admitted to being sexually active but had no history of sexually transmitted diseases (STDs).

On physical examination, she was alert and oriented. Her vital signs were normal with a temperature of 38.5°C, a pulse rate of 80 beats/min, and blood pressure (BP) of 130/80 mmHg. A general examination was unremarkable except for slight nuchal rigidity. Her throat was clear, and there was no lymphadenopathy. A pelvic examination revealed extensive vesicular and ulcerative lesions on the left labia minora and majora with marked edema. The cervix had exophytic (outward-growing) necrotic ulcerations. Specimens were taken to culture for Neisseria gonorrhoeae, viruses, and Chlamydia trachomatis.

General laboratory tests were unremarkable. The VDRL test was negative. A lumbar puncture was done. The opening pressure was normal. The cerebrospinal fluid (CSF) showed a mild pleocytosis with a leukocyte (WBC) count of 41/mm^3 with 21% polymorphonuclear leukocytes (PMNs) and 79% mononuclear cells, a glucose level of 46 mg/dl, and a protein level of 68 mg/dl (slightly elevated). The CSF VDRL test was negative. Cultures were sent. A rapid diagnostic test was done, which gave positive results. Cultures from the genital lesions and CSF verified the diagnosis 2 days later. By that time her condition had improved after 2 days of intravenous therapy. She was discharged home on oral medication.

1. What is the differential diagnosis of ulcerative genital lesions? Which rapid test was used so that specific therapy could be started?

2. Which complication of her underlying illness did she develop?

3. Which specific treatment did she receive?

4. Is she at risk for recurrences? How should she be managed?

5. How would you counsel this patient about recurrences? About what other important issues should she be counseled?

DISCUSSION

1. The most likely diagnosis is genital herpes. Genital herpes lesions are painful, whereas lesions due to *Treponema pallidum* are usually painless. Genital infections due to *Haemophilus ducreyi* or lymphogranuloma venereum can result in painful or painless ulcers, respectively, but they often result in suppurative lymphadenopathy. The etiologic agent of genital herpes in 70 to 90% of cases is herpes simplex virus type 2 (HSV-2), and in 10 to 30% of cases it is HSV-1. This virus is an enveloped, double-stranded DNA virus. Because it is an enveloped virus, it is spread only by direct contact with contaminated secretions.

   The diagnosis of HSV infection can be confirmed by isolating the virus in tissue culture cells or by examining scrapings from suspect lesions for HSV antigens by using rapid immunofluorescence techniques.

2. She had local and systemic signs and symptoms consistent with first-episode genital herpes. Up to one-third of patients may develop aseptic meningitis as a complication of primary genital herpes, as occurred in this case. The specific meningeal symptoms she developed included fever, headache, photophobia, and stiff neck.

   In contrast to aseptic meningitis associated with genital HSV-2 infection, herpes encephalitis in adults and older children is a more severe illness and is most often due to HSV-1 infection. Herpes encephalitis is a rare, sporadic central nervous system (CNS) viral infection. Patients present with fever, headache, and encephalopathic findings such as altered consciousness, behavorial and speech disturbances, and focal or diffuse neurologic signs. Babies born to women with genital herpes may develop herpes encephalitis from newly acquired HSV-2 infection. It is not proven why certain patterns of CNS infections with either HSV-1 or HSV-2 result in different CNS manifestations. The age of the patient, the route of viral dissemination (e.g., neural versus hematogenous), preexisting immunity, and/or specific viral properties may be factors.

3. The specific therapy is the antiviral agent acyclovir, which has specific activity against HSV. Because of the severity of her episode and her complication of aseptic meningitis, she received intravenous acyclovir followed by oral acyclovir therapy.

4. As with all viruses in the herpesvirus group, latent infections occur. Reactivation of latent viral infections can lead to recurrences of clinical disease. Daily suppressive therapy with oral acyclovir can decrease the recurrence rate. Patients can be successfully managed for several years with suppressive acyclovir.

5. Recurrences of genital herpes are generally milder than the primary episode of disease. She should be counseled about her risk for transmitting this infection to sexual partners and newborns. She should also be counseled about her risk for other STDs (syphilis, human immunodeficiency virus [HIV] infection) and the use of barrier contraceptives. She should be advised to have annual Pap smears since her history of an STD puts her at increased risk for infection with human papillomavirus (HPV). Data, although controversial, suggest an association between infection with certain serotypes of HPV and the development of cervical cancer.

REFERENCES

Corey, L., K. H. Fife, J. K. Benedetti, C. A. Winter, A. Fahnlander, J. D. Connor, M. A. Hintz, and K. K. Holmes. 1983. Intravenous acyclovir for the treatment of primary genital herpes. *Ann. Intern. Med.* **98:**914–921.

Corey, L., and P. G. Spear. 1986. Infections with herpes simplex viruses. *N. Engl. J. Med.* **314:**686-691; 749–757.

The patient was an 18-month-old female who presented to the emergency room with fever, a diffuse rash (onset 5 days ago), and a swollen right hand. On examination she was irritable but alert. Her temperature was 39°C and her heart rate was increased at 180 beats/min. She had diffuse vesiculopustular lesions over her entire body, with some areas showing older, crusted lesions. She had cellulitis of the right hand manifested by marked erythema, swelling, and tenderness. There were no mouth lesions, the lungs were clear, and the liver and spleen were not enlarged. Laboratory data were significant only for leukocytosis with a WBC count of 15,800/mm^3 with 88% neutrophils. The chest radiograph was clear. A radiograph of the right hand showed only soft tissue swelling. The patient was treated with intravenous cefazolin. Improvement in the condition of her right hand was notable within 48 h. This patient had a systemic viral infection with a complication of bacterial superinfection (cellulitis).

1. This patient had a characteristic rash at various stages of evolution. What is the differential diagnosis? What was her underlying viral illness?

2. Which complications other than bacterial superinfection (as seen in this case) can be seen as a result of this viral infection?

3. Which specific antiviral therapy has recently been shown to be efficacious?

4. After acute primary infection with this virus, latent infection develops. Which illness may occur years later as a result of viral reactivation? How do the clinical manifestations of this reactivation infection differ from those of primary infection?

5. What are the hospital infection control issues related to this patient's illness?

DISCUSSION

1. The underlying viral illness was varicella (chickenpox).

   The differential diagnosis in this case includes impetigo (group A streptococcal infection), disseminated enteroviral infection, or disseminated
   HSV infection in a child with underlying skin disease (e.g., eczema). This
   child had no history of a preexisting dermatologic disorder.

   The finding of generalized vesicular, pustular, and crusted skin lesions
   at various stages of evolution is characteristic of varicella. This illness is
   due to primary infection with varicella-zoster virus (VZV), which is a
   member of the herpesvirus group. These are enveloped, double-stranded
   DNA viruses.

   The diagnosis of chickenpox is often made on the basis of clinical
   findings alone. For laboratory confirmation, the virus can be isolated but
   this is rarely requested because the virus grows slowly in tissue culture,
   often requiring 2 to 3 weeks for isolation. Rapid and sensitive immunofluorescence assays are available and can be performed on scrapings
   taken from vesicular lesions. A Tzanck test can be performed, but is
   insensitive. The Tzanck test detects multinuclear giant cells, a cell type
   characteristically seen with VZV and HSV infections.

2. Complications include varicella pneumonia, hepatitis, arthritis, glomerulonephritis, encephalitis, and cerebellar ataxia. In addition, secondary
   bacterial infections of the skin lesions, as was seen in this case (cellulitis of
   the right hand), can also occur. These bacterial infections are most commonly caused by gram-positive organisms. Reye's syndrome with encephalopathy, elevated transaminase levels, and elevated serum ammonia
   levels can occur in children with varicella or influenza who take aspirin.

3. Recent studies have shown that acyclovir is beneficial in treating varicella
   in both immunocompetent and immunocompromised children and
   adults with varicella.

4. Zoster (shingles) can occur later in life as a result of reactivation of VZV
   from latent infection in ganglia. Typically, skin lesions appear in a dermatomal distribution innervated by the specific dorsal root or extramedullary cranial ganglia where VZV had been latent. Pain often occurs with the
   rash and can persist even after the skin lesions heal. This complication is
   more common in elderly patients. Rarely, skin lesions disseminate beyond
   the primary dermatome involved. In immunosuppressed patients, however, complicating viremia can occur with dissemination to extradermatomal skin sites, lungs, liver, and central nervous system. This latter condition
   is called atypical disseminated zoster.

5. Patients with VZV infection, especially chickenpox, are very contagious. Persons without a history of chickenpox are susceptible. Chickenpox in adults can be more severe, with an increased incidence of complications. Hospitalized patients with chickenpox must be in respiratory isolation, and strict infection control measures regarding skin contact (hand-washing, use of gloves and gowns, etc.) must be implemented.

Hospital workers without a history of chickenpox or those already known to be seronegative for VZV should not come into contact with these patients.

REFERENCES

Balfour, H. H., J. M. Kelly, C. S. Suarez, R. C. Heussner, J. A. Englund, D. D. Crane, P. V. McGuirt, A. F. Clemmer, and D. M. Aeppli. 1990. Acyclovir treatment of varicella in otherwise healthy children. *J. Pediatr.* **116:**633–639.

Dunkle, L. M., A. M. Arvin, R. J. Whitely, H. A. Rotbart, H. M. Feder, S. Feldman, A. A. Gershon, M. L. Levy, G. F. Hayden, P. V. McGuirt, J. Harris, and H. H. Balfour, Jr. 1991. A controlled trial of acyclovir for chickenpox in normal children. *N. Engl. J. Med.* **325:**1539–1544.

Straus, S. E., J. M. Ostrove, G. Inchauspe, J. M. Felser, A. Freifeld, K. D. Croen, and M. H. Sawyer. 1988. Varicella-zoster virus infections. Biology, natural history, treatment and prevention. *Ann. Intern. Med.* **108:**221–237.

The patient was an 18-year-old female who presented to the ear, nose, and throat clinic complaining of hoarseness and difficulty in swallowing. She had a 1-week history of sore throat, fever, easy fatigability, and myalgia. Her examination was significant for enlarged tonsils touching at the midline with exudate present. Bilateral tender anterior and posterior cervical lymphadenopathy, as well as splenomegaly, was present. Her CBC showed a hematocrit (Hct) of 44% and a WBC count of 7,000/mm^3 with 40% neutrophils, 28% lymphocytes, 12% atypical lymphocytes, and 20% monocytes. Liver function tests showed an aspartate aminotransferase (AST) level of 155 U/liter, an alanine aminotransferase (ALT) level of 208 U/liter, and an alkaline phosphatase level of 189 U/liter. Electrolytes were normal. Lateral neck radiographs showed a clear airway; the chest radiograph was negative. She was admitted to the hospital. A throat culture was sent to rule out gonococcal infection and beta-hemolytic streptococci. Viral serologies were ordered. She was admitted and treated with intravenous hydration, clindamycin, and steroids. On the second hospital day, a laboratory test confirmed her diagnosis. The clindamycin therapy was stopped, and p.o. prednisone was given. Her condition showed some improvement with decreased tonsillar size evident on examination by the fifth hospital day.

1. What was the differential diagnosis?

2. What was the specific etiology of her infection?

3. How might she have acquired this infection?

4. Which complications can this virus cause in immunosuppressed patients?

5. Why was this patient given steroids?

DISCUSSION

1. The differential diagnosis includes infectious mononucleosis, usually due to either Epstein-Barr virus (EBV) or cytomegalovirus (CMV), streptococcal pharyngitis, retropharyngeal abscess, gonococcal pharyngitis, and toxoplasmosis.

   This patient had EBV infection manifested by pharyngitis, tonsillitis, lymphadenopathy, splenomegaly, and lymphocytosis with atypical lymphocytes present.

2. Both the heterophile antibody assay and specific EBV serologic tests gave positive results in this patient and are indicative of acute EBV infection. Heterophile antibodies (to sheep erythrocytes) are present in 90% of EBV patients at some time during acute illness.

   The heterophile antibody test is helpful when positive. The test is highly sensitive in adolescents and adults, although less so in children younger than 4 years. If the heterophile antibody test is negative and the clinical suspicion for EBV-induced mononucleosis is high, specific EBV serologic tests should be done since a small number of EBV infections can be heterophile negative. CMV can also cause a heterophile-negative acute mononucleosis syndrome, so CMV serologic tests should also be done in heterophile-negative individuals.

3. EBV is acquired by intimate oral contact such as kissing. EBV replicates in oropharyngeal epithelial cells and is shed from this site in saliva for weeks to months after the onset of disease. EBV can be cultured from oropharyngeal washings or from circulating lymphocytes. However, these diagnostic procedures have little clinical utility because asymptomatic shedding of virus occurs in both healthy persons and those with unrelated illnesses. Sexual transmission of EBV has also been reported. Acquisition of EBV by blood transfusion or organ transplantation is also possible.

4. In immunosuppressed patients, especially patients with impaired cell-mediated immunity, EBV infection can result in a severe mononucleosislike illness which can be fatal. It can also lead to diffuse lymphoproliferative disorders including malignant lymphoma.

   Rare complications in otherwise normal hosts include pneumonia, central nervous system syndromes (encephalitis, Guillain-Barré syndrome), myocarditis, hepatitis, and aplastic anemia.

5. Steroids have been shown to be useful in reducing severe tonsillar enlargement which could lead to airway obstruction. They may also be useful in treating severe EBV-induced thrombocytopenia or hemolytic anemia. No specific antiviral therapy is available.

REFERENCES

Evans, A. S. 1978. Infectious mononucleosis and related syndromes. *Am. J. Med. Sci.* **276:**325–339.

Schooley, R. T., and R. Dolin. 1990. Epstein-Barr virus (infectious mononucleosis), p. 1172–1185. *In* G. L. Mandell, R. G. Douglas, Jr., and J. E. Bennett (ed.), *Principles and Practice of Infectious Diseases,* 3rd ed. Churchill Livingstone, Inc., New York.

The patient was a 1-year-old male admitted to the hospital in December because of fever and dehydration. His parents reported that he had a 1-day history of fever, diarrhea, emesis, and decreased urine output. On admission, his vital signs revealed a temperature of 39.5°C, slight tachycardia with a pulse of 126 beats/min, and respirations of 32/min. He was very somnolent. His general physical examination was remarkable only for hyperactive bowel sounds. Laboratory tests showed a leukocytosis with a WBC count of 14,200/mm^3 with 80% PMNs. Urinalysis was significant for a high specific gravity and ketones (consistent with the patient's dehydration). Stool, blood, and urine samples were sent for culture. A stool sample was also checked for ova and parasites. There were no fecal leukocytes. The patient was given intravenous normal saline and had nothing by mouth. Over the next 48 h his emesis abated. Once he was rehydrated and was tolerating oral feedings, he was discharged home. All routine cultures gave negative results, but a rapid viral diagnostic test was positive.

1. What is the differential diagnosis?

2. What is the most common cause of pediatric gastroenteritis? Briefly outline the pathophysiology seen with this organism. Is there any seasonality to this infection?

3. What rapid diagnostic test was used?

4. Which treatment is effective?

5. What special infection control precautions are necessary in the hospital setting when caring for a patient with gastroenteritis?

DISCUSSION

1. The differential diagnosis for acute diarrhea includes bacterial, parasitic, and viral etiologies of gastroenteritis. Because of the absence of fecal leukocytes, agents of invasive diarrhea such as *Salmonella, Shigella,* and *Campylobacter* spp. and *Entamoeba histolytica* are less likely, although certainly possible. The leading parasitic possibilities include *Giardia* and *Cryptosporidium* spp., especially if this child was in a day-care center. The viruses that can cause gastroenteritis include rotavirus (most frequent), enteric coronaviruses and unclassified small round viruses, Norwalk and Norwalk-like viruses, enteric adenovirus, calicivirus, and astrovirus. Vomiting is frequently seen in viral gastroenteritis and less frequently in infections with the other agents listed, making a viral agent much more likely in this particular case.

2. Group A rotavirus is the most common diarrheal pathogen seen in children less than 5 years old in the United States. The clinical spectrum varies from asymptomatic infection to severe, fatal disease. This virus causes a malabsorptive diarrhea, which can be reduced by stopping oral feedings. Vomiting, however, can remain a problem. The virus causes a blunting and atrophy of small intestinal villi, which results in reduced absorptive capacity. Although the disease can be severe and is occasionally fatal, especially in the malnourished, it generally is self-limited, lasting approximately 1 week in most cases. This disease is often referred to as "winter vomiting disease." It may be responsible for as many as 50% of pediatric hospitalizations during the winter. Characteristically, rotavirus illness occurs sporadically and not in widespread outbreaks. Norwalk virus infections can result in community outbreaks of diarrheal illness. Group B rotavirus has caused a large outbreak of diarrheal disease in Chinese adults, but is very uncommon in the United States.

3. The enzyme immunoassay (EIA) for rotavirus antigen was positive. This test and latex agglutination are the most common tests used to detect rotavirus. The virus was first discovered in the stools of children with vomiting and diarrhea by using electron microscopy. It was named for its characteristic wheellike ("rota") morphologic appearance on electron microscopy. However, this technique is not routinely used because of the ease of EIA and latex agglutination. RNA gel electrophoresis can also be used to detect rotavirus in stool specimens, but its use is primarily as a research tool for epidemiologic and vaccine studies. Virus isolation is not routinely performed in a clinical laboratory setting because it is inefficient and too time consuming.

4. Effective treatment to date includes aggressive use of intravenous and/or oral rehydration therapy. Oral rehydration is limited to patients without severe vomiting. There is no specific antiviral agent for rotavirus infections. Vaccines for prevention or modification of rotavirus-induced diarrhea are under development.

5. Strict hand-washing and the use of gloves by health care workers delivering care to patients with gastroenteritis are necessary. Hospital outbreaks of rotavirus infection have occurred when health care workers have transmitted the virus from one patient to another.

REFERENCE

Fairchild, P.G., and N. R. Blacklow. 1988. Viral diarrhea. *Infect. Dis. Clin. N. Am.* 2:677–684.

CASE 58

The patient was a 32-year-old male who presented to the emergency room with a 3-day history of fever (maximum temperature, 40°C), malaise, and back pain. Laboratory data revealed a WBC count of 4,700/mm^3 and abnormal liver function test results. Blood cultures were done and were subsequently reported as negative. He developed anorexia and jaundice in addition to fevers and malaise. He denied a history of intravenous drug use, sexual contact (for 2 months), and transfusions. Five weeks ago he was visiting friends in New York City, and they ate raw oysters. Recent telephone contact with one of the friends revealed that he had a similar illness.

On examination the patient was mildly icteric (jaundiced). There was no rash or lymphadenopathy. The abdominal examination revealed a tender liver, which was slightly enlarged. The spleen tip was nonpalpable. Laboratory tests showed an AST level of 2,501 U/liter, an alkaline phosphatase level of 298 U/liter, a bilirubin level of 2.2 mg/dl, and a lactate dehydrogenase (LDH) level of 1,102 U/liter. Blood was sent for diagnostic testing. Over the next month his symptoms resolved and the liver function test results returned to within normal limits.

1. A number of liver function tests were performed on this patient. What did they reveal? What was the differential diagnosis?

2. What was the etiology of his illness? How did he contract this infection?

3. What is the spectrum of disease associated with this organism?

4. How is this infection typically diagnosed?

5. How can infections with this agent be prevented?

DISCUSSION

1. This patient had extremely elevated liver enzyme levels, indicating that he had hepatitis. Given his case history, it is likely that his hepatitis was of an infectious etiology. The differential diagnosis of infectious hepatitis includes infection with hepatitis A, B, D (delta), and non-A, non-B (C, E) viruses, Epstein-Barr virus, and cytomegalovirus, toxoplasmosis, leptospirosis, and secondary syphilis. Noninfectious (e.g., drug-induced, alcoholic) hepatitis, cirrhosis, hepatic tumor, and abscess may also result in elevated liver enzyme levels and should also be considered in his differential diagnosis.

2. This patient had hepatitis A virus (HAV) infection. HAV is a single-stranded RNA virus belonging to the picornavirus group. It can survive readily in a variety of environments, including seawater. It is spread by the fecal-oral route and is well known to be acquired by eating raw oysters harvested from fecally contaminated water. Filter-feeding shellfish such as oysters, clams, and mussels are believed to concentrate the virus. This patient's history of eating raw oysters 5 weeks prior to the development of hepatitis symptoms is consistent with the incubation period for this virus, which is 2 to 8 weeks.

3. Acute HAV and HBV infections are clinically indistinguishable. HAV infection, as was seen in this case, is generally a benign, self-limited disease. Fulminant hepatitis has been reported with this virus, but is rare. Unlike HBV, HAV does not cause chronic infection and carrier states, nor is it associated with increased risk for hepatic carcinoma.

4. The diagnosis of HAV infection is frequently made on clinical grounds alone or as a diagnosis of exclusion; i.e., the patient has negative tests for HBV and HCV. The laboratory diagnosis is a serologic one in which the serum is examined for the presence of anti-HAV immunoglobulin M (IgM) antibodies. The detection of IgM antibodies is necessary because the presence of IgG antibodies to HAV indicates a previous infection at any time in the past. The virus is not cultivable by standard laboratory methods, nor is direct detection of the virus by immunologic or electron-microscopic techniques widely available.

5. Because HAV is usually obtained by ingestion of fecally contaminated food or water, good hygiene practices can usually prevent spread of this infection. Since HAV is frequently associated with ingestion of raw shellfish, eating only adequately cooked seafood will eliminate the risk since the virus is inactivated by boiling for 1 min. In outbreak situations, immune globulin is valuable in preventing or suppressing HAV infection.

Immune globulin is also given to nonimmune individuals (e.g., Peace Corps workers, missionaries, soldiers, and some tourists) who are traveling to areas of high endemicity which have poor sanitation. Protection in this situation usually lasts for 6 months, and people who remain in these areas for longer than 6 months must receive doses of immune globulin at 6-month intervals.

There are no commercially available HAV vaccines. However, clinical trials are under way to determine the safety and efficacy of candidate HAV vaccines.

REFERENCE

Wanke, C. A., and R. L. Guerrant. 1987. Viral hepatitis and gastroenteritis transmitted by shellfish and water. *Infect. Dis. Clin. N. Am.* **1:**649–664.

The patient was a 71-year-old farmer who presented to his doctor with a 3-month history of skin lesions on his lower legs. These lesions started as red spots, which then became necrotic and pustular. Two months previously, a biopsy revealed a vasculitis. One week prior to admission, he developed swelling of his left leg with fever and purulent drainage. He denied any trauma to his leg and had no shaking chills.

His medical history was significant for an illness 2 years ago characterized by generalized weakness, malaise, jaundice, and nausea. This illness lasted 2 months. He had no history of transfusions, but had been receiving acupuncture treatments for osteoarthritis in his neck. He was on no medication.

His physical examination was generally unremarkable except for the lower-extremity findings. There was no hepatosplenomegaly. Liver function tests revealed a leukocytosis with a WBC count of 12,800/mm^3 with 68% PMNs, 22% lymphocytes, 8% monocytes, and 2% eosinophils. Laboratory tests revealed an AST level of 33 U/liter, an ALT level of 22 U/liter, an alkaline phosphatase level of 17 U/liter, and a total biliribin level which was slightly elevated at 1.7 mg/dl. His hepatitis B surface antigen (HBsAg) test was positive, and his anti-HBs antibody test was negative.

The patient was treated with intravenous (i.v.) oxacillin, bed rest, and leg elevation. Cultures from the purulent drainage from his skin lesions revealed *Staphylococcus aureus*. Blood cultures were negative. He responded well to treatment with antistaphylococcal antibiotics.

1. This patient has a primary infectious process with a rare complication of vasculitis, which resulted in skin lesions that became secondarily infected. His primary infectious process can be attributed to which agent? Explain the significance of the HBsAg and anti-HBs results in this patient.

2. What is the relationship between his primary infecting agent and his development of vasculitis?

3. How do you think this patient contracted his infection? Name four common modes of transmission of this virus.

4. How can this infection be prevented in the general population? How can it be prevented in health professionals?

5. Which other virus can cause superinfection in patients with this virus?

6. What are other complications of infection with this agent, besides coinfection?

DISCUSSION

1. This patient's medical history suggests that 2 years previously he had contracted hepatitis. Hepatitis B virus (HBV) serologic tests done on this patient at admission indicate that he is chronically infected with HBV. In typical cases of HBV infection, acutely ill patients have a serologic profile similar to that of this patient, i.e., a positive HBsAg test and a negative anti-HBs test, but patients with acute infection often have elevated liver enzyme levels. As patients convalesce and their acute infection resolves, HBsAg declines, anti-HBs levels appear in almost all patients (99%), and liver enzyme levels return to normal. A small percentage (approximately 1%) of patients become chronically infected. Patients can develop chronic, active disease in which damage continues to the liver, as indicated by the continued elevation of liver enzyme levels, and they have the serologic profile seen in this patient. Alternatively, they can become chronic carriers of the virus. These individuals generally have liver enzyme levels within normal limits. Because this patient had surface antigen and normal liver enzyme levels, it is likely that he is a chronic carrier of HBV.

2. The patient also had vasculitis. Vasculitis is often due to deposition of immune complexes on blood vessel walls. His vasculitis may have been due to HBV-derived immune complexes, but that could be proven only by examining the diseased vessels for these immune complexes. This type of testing is not routinely available.

3. HBV can be spread parenterally as well as by sexual transmission. Infected mothers can also transmit virus to their newborn infants. Blood and body fluids can be the source of infectious virus. HBV infection can be acquired following percutaneous inoculation of virus using needles contaminated with blood or blood products. Thus groups at high risk include health care workers, hemodialysis patients, and intravenous drug abusers.

    It is well known that persons can acquire HBV from tattoos and acupuncture. Tattoo artists and acupuncturists notoriously lack proper sterilization practices. HBV is quite stable in the environment. Transmission via contaminated toothbrushes and razors can also occur.

    Although it is speculative, the only "at-risk" behavior in this patient's history is the fact that he received acupuncture treatments. This may be how he acquired hepatitis.

4. An HBV vaccine is available for use in the general population. In addition, individuals at high risk for parenteral or sexual spread of the virus should be appropriately counseled. Intravenous drug users should be instructed not to share needles and should clean their needles with bleach between uses. Condom use should be encouraged in individuals with multiple

sexual partners, and anal intercourse should be discouraged because of the increased risk due to tearing of rectal tissue with a concomitant exposure to blood.

Health care workers who may come in contact with blood should be vaccinated, should exercise care when using sharp objects, should protect themselves from mucous membrane exposure to blood, and should never recap needles or other sharp objects. Sharp objects should be disposed of properly to prevent secondary accidental wounds. All these preventive measures, with the exception of HBV vaccination, will also prevent the acquisition of HIV and other blood-borne infectious agents.

5. Patients with HBV infection are at risk for liver injury due to hepatitis delta virus (HDV). HDV is a defective RNA virus, so its replication requires coinfection with HBV. Exacerbations of hepatitis can occur in HBV carriers if they acquire HDV. This man is only theoretically at risk since the prevalence of HDV superinfections in the United States is low. The major risk groups for HDV infection are intravenous drug abusers and recipients of multiple transfusions (e.g., hemophiliacs).

6. Some of the hepatic complications of HBV infection include chronic hepatitis and the development of hepatocellular carcinoma. Extrahepatic complications are rare and include vasculitis (especially polyarteritis nodosa) and membranous glomerulonephritis. These two complications are most probably due to HBsAg-anti HBs immune complexes. Another rare complication is aplastic anemia, which can occur during acute infection.

REFERENCE

Robinson, W. S. 1990. Hepatitis B virus and hepatitis delta virus, p. 1204–1231. *In* G. L. Mandell, R. G. Douglas, Jr., and J. E. Bennett (ed.), *Principles and Practice of Infectious Diseases*, 3rd ed. Churchill Livingstone, Inc., New York.

CASE 60

The patient was a 3½-month-old male who presented in August with a 2-week history of diarrhea which abated with oral rehydration. One week later, he developed a fever with a temperature of 39.2°C and respiratory symptoms. He was found to have some wheezing and right otitis media. He was treated with Pediazole for presumed *Chlamydia* infection. He continued to have fever and developed irritability and vomiting. He returned to the clinic and was admitted.

On physical examination he was irritable and had a temperature of 36.6°C. He had tachycardia with a pulse of 180 beats/min. His blood pressure was normal. His fontanelles were normal. His neck was supple. His tympanic membranes were dull and distorted bilaterally. The rest of his examination was unremarkable. Laboratory tests showed an anemia with a hemoglobin level of 10.4 g/dl; the WBC count was 9,300/mm³ with 60% lymphocytes. Electrolyte levels were normal. A lumbar puncture was done, and CSF revealed a WBC count of 75/mm³ with 72% neutrophils, 8% lymphocytes, and 20% monocytes; the glucose level was 60 mg/dl and the protein level was 22 mg/dl (both normal). A Gram stain was negative for bacteria, and few PMNs were present.

CSF bacterial antigen testing was done for *Haemophilus influenzae, Streptococcus pneumoniae,* group B streptococci, and *Neisseria meningitidis.* These tests were negative. CSF samples were sent for viral cultures. Intravenous ceftriaxone and ampicillin were begun empirically for presumed bacterial meningitis. One day later his fontanelle was full. A head computed tomogram (CT) scan was normal. On the second hospital day his condition had improved and his anterior fontanelle was less full. Blood, urine, and CSF bacterial cultures were negative. He was discharged on the fourth hospital day to complete a 10-day course of intramuscular ceftriaxone on an outpatient basis.

After discharge, his CSF viral culture became positive.

1. Does this patient have meningitis? Explain your answer.

2. Which type of virus is likely to be causing this infection?

3. Describe the transmission and pathogenesis of infection with viruses of this group.

4. Give some examples of specific clinical syndromes associated with particular virus serotypes in this group.

5. Describe the treatment and prevention of these viral infections.

DISCUSSION

1. The finding of >3 white blood cells/mm^3 of CSF is abnormal and is indicative of meningitis. The patient was treated for bacterial meningitis because of the predominance of neutrophils in the CSF. Early in the course of viral meningitis (the first 24 to 48 h), neutrophils can be predominant. However, mononuclear cells are predominant later in the disease. The normal CSF glucose level also argues against bacterial meningitis. This CSF picture may also be seen in mycobacterial and fungal meningitis, both of which would be very unusual in an immunocompetent infant. Finally, a positive CSF viral culture confirms the diagnosis of viral meningitis.

2. Viruses of the enterovirus group (coxsackievirus, echovirus, and poliovirus) characteristically cause this type of illness during late summer and early fall. Because of poliovirus vaccine usage, it is most likely that this patient had infection due to either coxsackievirus or echovirus. These are single-stranded RNA viruses known as picornaviruses. This patient's viral culture was positive for coxsackievirus.

3. Enteroviruses are transmitted mostly by the fecal-oral route, but some serotypes may be spread by respiratory secretions or fomites.
   Enteroviruses are acid stable; after replication in the oropharynx they can survive transit through the stomach. Replication then occurs in the lower intestinal tract. Following replication in the lymphoid tissue of the gastrointestinal tract, the viruses can pass to the bloodstream. Spread to the liver, spleen, lymph nodes, and specific target organs (meninges, heart, and skin) can result.

4. All three types of enteroviruses can cause aseptic meningitis. The incidence is highest in children less than 1 year old, such as this patient. Myocarditis, pericarditis, and pleurodynia are associated with group B coxsackievirus. Polioviruses characteristically cause paralysis (usually asymmetric). Herpangina (vesicular oral ulcers) and hand-foot-and-mouth disease are classically caused by group A coxsackieviruses. A variety of coxsackieviruses and echoviruses have been associated with benign viral exanthems, mimicking measles or rubella.

5. The management of patients with enteroviral infections includes supportive care. Infection control measures are recommended for patients and their families to interrupt transmission of virus to others who may be susceptible. These include hand-washing. This is of particular importance in day-care centers, where agents that are spread by the fecal-oral route (HAV, *Giardia* spp., *Shigella* spp., etc.) are of particular concern.

Specific antiviral therapy is not available. Vaccines, both attenuated oral and inactivated preparations, are available for the prevention of poliovirus infections (see case 61).

REFERENCE

Modlin, J. F., and J. S. Kinney. 1987. Perinatal enteroviral infections, p. 57–78. *In* S. C. Aronoff, W. T. Hughes, S. Kohl, W. T. Speck, and E. R. Wald (ed.), *Advances in Pediatric Infectious Diseases*, vol. 2. Mosby-Year Book, Chicago.

This 12-year-old male, who had been in apparent good health, complained of an occipital headache 4 days prior to admission. Three days prior to admission he complained of weakness in his lower extremities. On that day he was hospitalized at an outside hospital; he complained of a stiff neck and underwent a lumbar puncture (results unavailable). The patient noted weakness in his left arm, and prior to his transfer to our hospital his left arm was flail and he had difficulty talking. He also complained of epigastric pain and soreness of his neck.

On examination, the patient was in acute respiratory distress with grunting respirations and a high respiratory rate of 42/min. He was tachycardic and normotensive. Examination was remarkable for an abnormal neurologic response. The patient was very fatigued, could count only to 8, and could not blow air. Cranial nerves I to VII were intact. The patient was hoarse. He could move his tongue and could open his mouth poorly. The patient had no movement of his left arm. He had decreased strength of his right triceps, biceps, and hand muscles. He had decreased strength of his hamstrings and weakness in flexion and extension of his left leg (more severe than that of the right). No deep tendon reflexes were elicited. The patient had no sensory or vibratory sensation. A lumbar puncture revealed a pleocytosis with a WBC count of $58/mm^3$ (2% polymorphonuclear cells and 98% lymphocytes). CSF glucose and protein levels were normal. His immunization history was questionable.

Blood, CSF, and stool specimens were sent to the diagnostic virology laboratory. A virus culture of the stool specimen revealed the diagnosis.

1. Which virus was isolated from the patient's stool culture?

2. Describe the epidemiology of this infection. In the vaccine era, what are the risk factors for infection with this virus?

3. For which cell types does this virus have specific tropism? Describe the pathogenesis of infection.

4. How is infection managed (prevented and treated)?

DISCUSSION

1. Poliovirus type 1 was isolated from the patient's stool specimen. This is an enterovirus belonging to a large group of viruses known as picornaviruses (small RNA viruses). There are three poliovirus serotypes: poliovirus types 1, 2, and 3.

2. This virus is transmitted by the fecal-oral route similar to other enteroviruses. Prior to the widespread use of vaccination, infections resulted in epidemics usually in the summer months. Salk developed the first successful vaccine, which was an inactivated poliovirus vaccine (IPV). Later, Sabin developed a live attenuated oral polio vaccine (OPV). The oral vaccine strain replicates in the gastrointestinal tract and can be shed in the feces. Poliovirus isolates of vaccine origin are occasionally recovered in fecal specimens of recently vaccinated individuals, but only rarely cause disease (see the discussion of question 4). Epidemic poliovirus disease no longer exists in the United States. Small outbreaks have been reported in isolated groups of unvaccinated persons, however. Isolated cases can occur in unvaccinated family contacts of recently immunized children.

3. Poliovirus replicates in the gastrointestinal tract, can cause viremia, and infects primarily the motor and autonomic neurons. The major sites of infection are the anterior horn cells of the spinal cord and the motor nuclei of the brain stem.

   The disease spectrum ranges from asymptomatic viral shedding to severe paralytic poliomyelitis. Symptoms and signs of aseptic meningitis (headache, photophobia, stiff neck) can develop. When paralysis develops, the most characteristic feature is the asymmetrical distribution. Patients who are immunodeficient are more predisposed to poliovirus infections.

   This patient developed spinal and bulbar poliomyelitis. Bulbar polio is due to paralysis of muscles innervated by the cranial nerves. Most complications of paralytic poliomyelitis are respiratory. Myocarditis and gastrointestinal complications can also occur.

4. The most commonly used vaccine for preventing polio is the OPV. The IPV is preferred for immunodeficient persons and for unvaccinated adults, however, because clinical infection may develop following ingestion of the OPV.

   Specific antiviral agents for polio are not available. Management is focused largely on supportive care.

REFERENCE

LaForce, F. M. 1990. Poliomyelitis vaccines: success and controversy. *Infect. Dis. Clin. N. Am.* **4**:75–83.

The patient was a 59-year-old female who underwent a cardiac transplant 6 months earlier for an idiopathic cardiomyopathy. Since the transplant she has done reasonably well, with the exception of two episodes of acute rejection which required increased doses of steroids to control rejection. One week prior to this admission, she complained of malaise, fatigue, a low-grade fever, and mild dyspnea on exertion. She was admitted to determine the etiology of her complaints. The physical examination was significant only for a temperature of 38.3°C and cushingoid body habitus (due to the steroids). Examination of her lungs revealed fine bibasilar rales. A stool specimen was guaiac positive. Her laboratory studies revealed a hematocrit of 24% (normal, 33 to 35%), a WBC count of 2,300/mm^3 (leukopenia), and a normal platelet count. She was transfused with 3 units of blood and underwent upper gastrointestinal endoscopy, which revealed nodular gastric erosions. Biopsies and brushings were taken and submitted to the pathology and microbiology laboratories. A chest radiograph revealed diffuse infiltrates. A bronchoscopy was done, and transbronchial biopsy and bronchoalveolar lavage specimens were sent for histopathologic and cytologic examination and bacterial, fungal, viral, and acid-fast bacillus (AFB) culture. Gram stains were negative. The next day, hematoxylin and eosin (H&E) stains of the gastric lesion brushings, as well as the lung tissue, revealed the source of her infection. Viral cultures were positive 2 weeks later, confirming the diagnosis.

1. Which opportunistic infectious agents can cause pneumonitis and gastritis? What was the most likely etiology of her infection?

2. Which other two types of patient populations are subject to serious infections with this virus?

3. Which clinical manifestations are caused by this virus other than fever, leukopenia, gastritis, and pneumonitis?

4. This patient and her donor were seropositive for this virus. What are all of the likely sources of her infection?

5. Which other opportunistic infections might she develop?

6. Which specimens other than tissue should be sent for viral culture?

DISCUSSION

1. Cytomegalovirus (CMV) is the most common infectious agent complicating transplantation. CMV can cause both pneumonia and gastritis. Other opportunistic infectious agents that can cause both pneumonia and gastritis include herpes simplex virus (as a result of virus spread down nasogastric or nasopharyngeal tubes), *Histoplasma capsulatum*, *Cryptococcus* spp., *Mucor* spp., and *Aspergillus* spp. All of these infectious agents except CMV rarely cause these complications.

2. In addition to transplant recipients, AIDS patients and newborns can develop severe CMV infections. AIDS patients have a high incidence of CMV retinitis, which is rarely seen in transplant patients. The CMV pneumonia that transplant patients develop usually is more severe than that seen in AIDS patients. The reasons for different patterns of CMV disease in these high-risk populations are unclear.

   Congenital CMV infection can result in deafness, psychomotor retardation, chorioretinitis, pneumonia, hepatitis, and rash.

3. CMV can cause fever, infectious mononucleosis-like syndromes, leukopenia and complicating opportunistic infections, thrombocytopenia, hepatitis, esophagitis, gastritis, cholangitis, chorioretinitis, and pneumonia. It can cause adrenalitis, skin rash, and central nervous system infection, but these are rare.

4. Transplant recipients who are CMV seropositive pretransplant are at risk for developing reactivation of their own latent CMV infection and consequently symptoms of CMV disease. If these patients receive transplants from CMV-seropositive donors, they are also at risk for infection with the donor virus strain. Another source of CMV infection is transfused blood. CMV-seronegative transplant recipients who receive CMV-seropositive organs are at risk for developing primary infections. These patients tend to have more frequent and more severe disease episodes than do CMV-seropositive recipients whose own virus is reactivated.

5. Other opportunistic infections in cardiac transplant recipients include those caused by pathogens common in patients with impaired cell-mediated immunity. These infections include toxoplasmosis, *Pneumocystis carinii* pneumonia, varicella zoster, cryptococcal pneumonia or meningitis, *Listeria monocytogenes* bacteremia or meningitis, and *Nocardia* spp. pneumonia.

6. Specimens of respiratory secretions, urine, and blood for buffy coat (i.e., white blood cells, especially neutrophils) cultures should be sent to the diagnostic laboratory for virus isolation. Biopsy specimens of involved tissue can also be submitted to the laboratory. CMV can be detected by

finding characteristic cytopathic effects in infected fibroblast tissue culture cells or by detection of CMV antigen in a rapid shell vial culture amplification system. Positive CMV urine culture in the absence of positive test results from buffy coat or respiratory secretion specimens should be interpreted cautiously since asymptomatic shedding of CMV in urine may occur in immunosuppressed patients. Monoclonal antibodies to CMV can be used for the direct detection of CMV antigens by immunofluorescence by using buffy coat preparations of white blood cells or tissues obtained by biopsy or autopsy. Cytomegalic cells, characteristically with "owls' eye" nuclei, can also be seen directly in histopathologic examination of tissue biopsy specimens, as was the case for this patient.

REFERENCES

Gentry, L. O., and B. Zeluff. 1988. Infection in the cardiac transplant patient, p. 623–648. *In* R. H. Rubin and L. S. Young (ed.), *Clinical Approach to Infection in the Compromised Host*, 2nd ed. Plenum Publishing Corp., New York.

Hofflin, J. M., I. Potasman, J. C. Balwin, P. E. Oyer, E. B. Stinson, and J. S. Remington. 1987. Infectious complications in heart transplant recipients receiving cyclosporine and corticosteroids. *Ann. Intern. Med.* **106:**209–216.

The patient was a 9-year-old female who was brought to her pediatrician in February because of fever and rash for 2 days. She also had a headache, sore throat, and mild cough. There were no gastrointestinal symptoms. No one else in the household was ill, but she had a classmate with a similar illness.

On examination she was alert and in mild distress. Her temperature was 38.3°C, her pulse rate was 110 beats/min, her blood pressure was 90/60 mmHg, and her respiratory rate was 40/min. She had a mild conjunctivitis. Her posterior pharynx was injected, and petechiae were present on her soft palate. The buccal mucosa was injected with scattered raised papular lesions. She had a macular rash on her trunk, face, and arms. Her chest radiograph was normal. A throat swab was sent for culture, and blood was drawn for viral serologic examination. Subsequently, the throat culture was read as negative for group A beta-hemolytic streptococci. Acute- and convalescent-phase serum specimens (obtained 2 weeks later) revealed the diagnosis, and the school nurse was notified.

1. What is the differential diagnosis in an individual who presents with the symptoms cited in this case, with specific emphasis on the skin rash? What is the agent of this patient's infection?

2. How is the diagnosis of this infection usually made?

3. Describe the typical clinical course of this infection, and name three complications which can occur.

4. How can infection with this virus be prevented? Why has there been a recent resurgence in the number of cases?

5. How would you manage her case? Are specific treatments available?

DISCUSSION

1. In general, the differential diagnosis is quite large in patients with fever and rash, so it is important to focus on the specific type of rash. In this patient the rash was diffuse and macular. Macular or maculopapular rashes are seen with viruses such as measles virus, rubella virus, roseola virus, enteroviruses, EBV, CMV, and parvovirus B19. Other types of infections associated with this type of rash include meningococcal infection, salmonellosis, mycoplasma infection, Rocky Mountain spotted fever, secondary syphilis, and subacute bacterial endocarditis. Coexisting enanthemas (involvement of mucous membranes) can help to narrow down the diffential diagnosis. This patient had a rash that was readily recognizable (i.e., measles) from its specific appearance and accompanying findings of coryza, conjunctivitis, pharyngitis, and palatal petechiae. The measles virus is a paramyxovirus (a single-stranded RNA virus). Humans are the only natural host.

2. The diagnosis of measles is usually made on clinical grounds, with laboratory diagnostic procedures playing a secondary role. A nasopharyngeal aspirate stained with fluorescence-labeled antibody detects the measles virus directly in clinical specimens, allowing same-day laboratory diagnosis of infection.

    IgM-based tests are also available for the rapid diagnosis of measles. Serum samples for IgM tests should be collected after day 3 of the rash since IgM antibody may not be detectable before this time. The virus can be isolated in tissue culture, but isolation is difficult and unreliable for the diagnosis of measles.

3. After exposure, the incubation period of measles is 10 to 14 days. Typically, patients initially develop fever, cough, coryza, conjunctivitis, sore throat, and headaches. Several days later a generalized morbilliform rash appears. Koplik spots, which are pathognomonic for measles, may be seen. These are small bluish-gray lesions on a red base, which appear on the buccal mucosa.

    The virus multiplies in the upper respiratory tract and conjunctiva. Viremia then develops, and after this viremia the patient experiences fever, constitutional symptoms, and rash. Leukopenia usually accompanies acute infection.

    In the upper respiratory tract, edema and loss of cilia as a result of the measles infection can predispose to secondary bacterial invasion. Complications of measles include bacterial pneumonia and otitis media. In the developing world, secondary diarrheal disease is often seen, especially in malnourished infants and children. The combination of these two diseases has a much higher mortality rate than does either disease alone. The mechanism by which measles predisposes to the acquisition of diarrheal pathogens is unknown.

The most severe complication is encephalitis, which develops in 1 of every 1,000 to 2,000 cases. This develops 1 to 14 days after the rash. A high proportion of patients with encephalitis are left with neurologic sequelae. Subacute sclerosing panencephalitis (SSPE) is an extremely rare complication of early infection and usually is seen in patients less than 2 years old. SSPE is a persistent encephalitic infection which is distinct from the encephalitis that may complicate acute measles infection. The virus which causes SSPE may be a defective measles virus or another measles virus variant. SSPE has an insidious onset, usually manifested by behavior problems. The disease progresses over a period of weeks to months, resulting in severe neurologic dysfunction including seizure activity, loss of motor function, coma, and eventually death.

4. Measles can be prevented with live attenuated vaccines. In addition to vaccination, infection may be prevented by the use of passive immunity (immunoglobulin). This is usually administered to persons at significant risk of severe measles following specific exposure. Immunoglobulin can be used in babies less than 1 year old and children with cancer and/or specific defects in cell-mediated immunity.

A recent increase in the number of measles cases (mostly in preschool and college-age groups) is due to failure to immunize persons, to primary vaccine failure, and to imported cases. This patient had a history of being vaccinated, and so she most probably represents a case of primary vaccine failure.

5. This patient should be managed with supportive therapy. No specific antiviral treatment is available. The school nurse and local health department should be notified about this case (as was done) as soon as possible so that control measures (vaccination programs, etc.) can be implemented.

REFERENCES

Peter, G. 1991. Measles immunization: recommendations, challenges and more information. *JAMA* **265**:2111–2112.

Weber, D. J., W. R. Gammon, and M. S. Cohen. 1990. The acutely ill patient with fever and rash, p. 479–489. *In* G. L. Mandell, R. G. Douglas, Jr., and J. E. Bennett (ed.), *Principles and Practice of Infectious Disease,* 3rd ed. Churchill Livingstone, Inc., New York.

This 34-year-old man was well until 3 days prior to admission, when he noted the onset of fever, weakness, fatigue, headache, sore throat, and a cough productive of white sputum. One day prior to admission he awakened with burning chest discomfort that was made worse by coughing and by deep breathing. He developed shortness of breath and was seen at a university infirmary, where he appeared acutely ill with a fever. A chest radiograph demonstrated bilateral infiltrates consistent with pneumonia. An arterial blood gas analysis, done while the patient was breathing room air, was notable for significant hypoxemia (pO_2, 48 mmHg; normal, 85 to 100 mmHg). The patient's shortness of breath increased markedly, and he was transferred to the hospital, where he was found to be cyanotic and febrile to 39.8°C and to have a respiratory rate of 44/min with labored respirations. His sputum was grossly bloody with apparent clumps of tissue. Examination of the sputum revealed a grossly bloody background, numerous neutrophils, and sheets of gram-positive cocci in clusters. Despite appropriate antibiotic therapy and maximal intensive care support, the patient died. His illness occurred during January.

1. The sputum Gram stain is most consistent with which bacterial pathogen?

2. In addition to the bacterial infection noted above, the nonspecific symptoms that began this illness and the time of year in which he became ill suggest a viral illness as well. Which viral illness is most likely?

3. How is the presence of these two processes related?

4. Which other bacterial causes of pneumonia can complicate this viral infection?

DISCUSSION

1. The presence of gram-positive cocci in clusters is strongly suggestive of staphylococci. The *Staphylococcus* species that causes severe, necrotic pneumonia is *Staphylococcus aureus*. The patient's physicians treated him with an antistaphylococcal antibiotic based on the result of the sputum Gram stain. Subsequent blood and sputum cultures were positive for *S. aureus*.

2. A febrile illness with this patient's initial symptoms and the time of year (January) are consistent with (but certainly not diagnostic of) an infection with influenza virus. Pharyngeal viral cultures obtained at the time of hospital admission as well as postmortem cultures were positive for influenza A virus. This patient had a primary influenza virus pneumonia complicated by a secondary bacterial pulmonary infection due to *Staphylococcus aureus*.

3. Staphylococcal pneumonia is an established complication of infection with influenza virus. In fact, the presence of an increased number of cases of *S. aureus* pneumonia may alert authorities to an otherwise unrecognized outbreak of influenza. One of the reasons for increased susceptibility to secondary bacterial infection is that the influenza virus induces a defect in the ciliary function of the respiratory tract. Studies have shown that the microtubular structure in ciliated epithelial cells is disrupted in individuals with influenza. This disruption adversely affects the function of cilia that is central to protecting the lungs from bacterial invaders.

4. Secondary bacterial pneumonia following (or simultaneous with) influenza virus infection is also caused by *Streptococcus pneumoniae* and *Haemophilus influenzae*. This is more likely to occur in elderly persons than in the young and adds considerably to the mortality in influenza epidemics.

REFERENCE

Carson, J. L., A. M. Collier, and S.-C. S. Hu. 1985. Acquired ciliary defects in nasal epithelium of children with acute viral upper respiratory infections. *N. Engl. J. Med.* **321**:463–468.

The patient was a 19-year-old pregnant female who presented at 22 weeks gestation with signs and symptoms of preeclampsia.

An ultrasonogram revealed intrauterine fetal demise. Hydrops (abnormal accumulation of fluid in tissues) was present. Induced labor and delivery were performed, and a stillborn female fetus was delivered. An autopsy was performed on the fetus, and severe autolysis was evident. This is consistent with intrauterine fetal demise. On histopathologic examination of the fetus, characteristic intranuclear viral inclusions were seen in erythroid precursor cells in the bone marrow and liver. Serologic evidence of acute infection due to maternal exposure to a virus supported the diagnosis for this case.

1. Describe the viral etiology in this case.

2. Name three modes of transmission of this infection.

3. Describe at least two of the other four clinical syndromes caused by infection with this virus.

4. Which laboratory tests are available for the diagnosis of this infection?

5. Which other viruses may be congenitally acquired?

DISCUSSION

1. This intrauterine fetal death was due to acute maternal infection with parvovirus B19, a single-stranded DNA virus.

2. Parvovirus B19 can be transmitted vertically from mother to fetus, as in this case. In addition, it is transmitted by the respiratory route and by transfusions. By early adulthood, 30 to 60% of the population have acquired parvovirus B19 infection. Parvovirus B19 infects and lyses erythroid precursor cells. This can lead to transient aplastic crises (TAC) in patients with hemolytic states. Bone marrow examinations in these patients characteristically show erythroid hypoplasia. The duration of TAC is usually 7 to 10 days. Fetal death appears to be caused by severe anemia. Fetal infections may not always be fatal. There is no association of parvovirus B19 with congenital anomalies.

3. In addition to asymptomatic infection, parvovirus B19 can cause erythema infectiosum. Erythema infectiosum (fifth disease) is a benign rash of childhood. Infected persons develop fever and facial erythema described as a "slapped cheek" appearance. A lacy reticular rash may occur on the trunk and extremities. An acute symmetrical peripheral arthritis in adults, TAC in patients with hemoglobinopathies (e.g., sickle cell disease), chronic anemia in immunodeficient patients, and intrauterine infection and fetal death are the other clinical syndromes caused by parvovirus B19.

4. The diagnosis can be made by demonstrating parvovirus B19 IgM serum antibodies or by the presence of parvovirus B19 DNA or antigen in the serum. Serologic testing for parvovirus antibodies is not widely available, and antigen and DNA detection of parvovirus are currently both experimental. Histopathologically, eosinophilic intranuclear inclusions in infected tissues or virus particles seen by electron microscopy can lead to the diagnosis. Although parvovirus B19 can replicate in bone marrow explant cultures, no routine virus isolation methods are currently available for diagnostic purposes.

5. Other viruses which can be congenitally acquired include rubella virus, cytomegalovirus, hepatitis B virus, HIV, HSV, VZV, enteroviruses, and adenovirus. Rubella virus and CMV characteristically cause teratogenic effects (congenital anomalies), whereas the remaining viruses cause disseminated infection and disease.

REFERENCES

Anderson, L. J., and E. S. Hurwitz. 1988. Human parvovirus B19 and pregnancy. *Clin. Perinatol.* **15:**273–286.

Frickhofen, N., A. Raghavachar, W. Hert, H. Heimpl, and B. J. Cohen. 1986. Human parvoviral infection. *N. Engl. J. Med.* **314:**646.

Thurn, J. 1988. Human parvovirus B19: historical and clinical review. *Rev. Infect. Dis.* **10:**1005–1011.

CASE 66

The patient was a 31-year-old male with severe hemophilia B. Two months prior to admission he developed malaise and a 15-lb (6.8-kg) weight loss. One week prior to admission he developed pain upon swallowing food and liquids. He had had a low-grade fever for one week. Two days prior to admission he developed rapidly progressive decreased vision in his right eye. The physical examination was significant for fever, tachycardia, and blood pressure of 140/72 mmHg. His fundoscopic examination revealed several characteristic hemorrhagic lesions described as "catsup on cottage cheese" in his right eye. His throat was erythematous, but there were no vesicles or whitish plaques. His laboratory tests revealed a hematocrit of 30%, WBC count of 4,100/mm^3, and 85,000 platelets. His chest radiograph was negative. An endoscopy was done, and pathologic tests showed findings specific to his diagnosis which explained his pain upon swallowing. Consultation with the Ophthalmology Department was obtained to evaluate his retinal lesions and visual changes.

1. The patient has infections caused by two different viruses. What are the two infections?

2. What laboratory tests are available for the diagnosis of the primary infectious agent?

3. What is the most common ocular complication in this patient population?

4. Which specific antiviral treatments should this patient receive?

5. Would you expect his T-helper (CD4$^+$) lymphocyte count to be greater than or less than 200/mm^3?

6. Are hemophiliacs born after 1990 at risk for this underlying viral infection?

253

DISCUSSION

1. This patient's primary infection was due to human immunodeficiency virus (HIV). He acquired this infection from multiple transfusions with clotting factor concentrates. These clotting factors are contained within a pooled concentrate obtained from multiple blood donors. Prior to the availability of a specific HIV antibody test used for screening blood donors, these pooled concentrates were often contaminated with HIV. Heat treatment (pasteurization) of clotting factor, instituted several years ago, has been shown to inactivate HIV.

   His secondary infection was with cytomegalovirus (CMV), which caused his retinitis and esophagitis.

2. A variety of techniques have been adapted for the detection of HIV. It should be emphasized that the detection of HIV in patients does not indicate that these patients have AIDS. AIDS is the terminal stage of HIV infection, usually occurring several years after primary infection. By this time, the virus has destroyed most of the protective capability of the T-helper cell arm of the immune system, putting the infected individual at risk for developing a wide variety of opportunistic infections and neoplastic processes.

   For the vast majority of patients, HIV infection is diagnosed by detecting antibodies to the virus in the patient's blood. Testing is done in two stages: a screening test and a confirmatory test if the screening test gives positive results. The screening test most frequently used in North America to detect HIV-1 is an EIA. If this test is positive it is repeated, and if it remains positive the confirmatory test is done. The confirmatory test is a Western immunoblot assay. In this test, HIV is disrupted and viral proteins are separated on polyacrylamide gels by a process known as electrophoresis. These separated proteins are transferred to a membrane, usually made of either nitrocellulose or nylon. A serum sample from the patient is incubated with these protein blots, and an assay is done to see whether the individual has antibodies which bind to specific HIV proteins. An individual is determined to be HIV positive if he or she has antibodies which react with two or more of the following viral glycoproteins: gp24, gp41, and gp120/gp160. Serologic diagnosis has several limitations. False-positive EIAs have been reported in multiparous women and individuals with autoimmune disease. In populations with a low incidence of HIV disease, false-positive EIA results may be more frequent than true-positive ones. Serologic tests often give negative results in the very early, acute phase of infection, and patients may take from several weeks to as long as 6 months before they become HIV positive serologically. Western blot techniques are technically demanding and are not available in many hospital laboratories. Finally, serologic testing cannot be used in children less than 15 months of age because positive results may reflect passively acquired maternal antibodies rather than the children's own.

Several methods that detect the virus directly in the patient's blood have been developed. They include p24 antigen, culture, and the polymerase chain reaction. These tests are used diagnostically either early in the disease course before an immune response has been mounted or in infants in whom the presence of antibodies may not be diagnostic.

3. CMV chorioretinitis is the most frequent ophthalmologic complication in patients with HIV infection. Other causes of retinitis in this population include toxoplasmosis, syphilis, and *Candida* infection. This latter infection is a problem primarily in intravenous drug users.

4. For the treatment of his HIV infection, he should receive the specific antiretroviral agent zidovudine (formerly known as AZT). If he becomes intolerant to zidovudine, he could receive dideoxyinosine (ddI). For treating his CMV retinitis and esophagitis, he should receive ganciclovir. Both zidovudine and ganciclovir can result in hematologic abnormalities, particularly neutropenia and anemia. It is very difficult to give these two drugs concurrently. Often the zidovudine must be withheld temporarily while the patient receives daily ganciclovir treatments. Usually after 14 to 21 days of ganciclovir induction, less frequent administrations are given during maintenance therapy. If maintenance ganciclovir therapy is stopped, this patient would be at high risk for relapse of his retinitis and, possibly, his esophagitis. Patients can sometimes be given zidovudine at lower doses at this stage. Another therapy for CMV retinitis is foscarnet, which can be combined with zidovudine more successfully than can ganciclovir.

5. Patients with advanced HIV disease and T-helper lymphocyte counts less than 100 cells/mm^3 are at the highest risk for developing CMV disease.

6. Because of HIV antibody testing of all blood donors and the routine pasteurization of clotting-factor concentrates, recently born hemophiliacs have significantly less risk of acquiring HIV.

Recent epidemiologic studies revealed that clotting factors are unlikely to transmit CMV. Hemophiliacs therefore are not significantly more likely to be CMV infected than are age-matched controls.

REFERENCES

Becherer, P. R., M. L. Smiley, T. J. Matthews, K. J. Weinhold, C. W. McMillan, and G. C. White. 1990. Human immunodeficiency virus-1 disease progression in hemophiliacs. *Am. J. Hematol.* **34**:204–209.

Bloom, J. N., and A. G. Palestine. 1988. The diagnosis of CMV retinitis. *Ann. Intern. Med.* **109:**963–969.

Schooley, R. T. 1990. Cytomegalovirus in the setting of infection with the human immunodeficiency virus. *Rev. Infect. Dis.* **12:**s811–s819.

Table 4. Medically important viruses

Enveloped DNA viruses	RNA viruses
Herpes simplex virus type 1	Polioviruses
Herpes simplex virus type 2	Coxsackieviruses
Epstein-Barr virus	Echoviruses
Varicella-zoster virus	Enteroviruses
Cytomegalovirus	Rhinoviruses
Human herpesvirus 6	Hepatitis A virus
Variola virus	Norwalk virus
Vaccinia virus	Rubella virus
	Eastern equine encephalitis virus
Nonenveloped DNA viruses	Western equine encephalitis virus
Hepatitis B virus	St. Louis encephalitis virus
Parvovirus B19	Hepatitis C virus
Human papillomaviruses	Hepatitis delta virus
JC virus	Dengue viruses
Adenovirus	Human coronavirus
	Rabies virus
RNA-containing retroviruses	Parainfluenza viruses
Human immunodeficiency virus types 1 and 2	Mumps virus
Human T-cell lymphotropic virus types I and II	Measles virus
	Respiratory syncytial virus
	Influenza A, B, and C viruses
Slow viruses	Rotavirus
Creutzfeldt-Jakob disease agent	
Kuru agent	
Scrapie agent	

Table 5. Table of normal values

WBC:	4,000–12,000/mm^3
Neutrophils:	2,000–7,500/mm^3
Eosinophils:	40–400/mm^3
Platelets:	150,000–400,000/mm^3
pO$_2$:	85–100 mmHg

	Male	Female
Hemoglobin:	13.4–17.4 mg/dl	12.3–15.7 mg/dl
Hematocrit:	40–54%	38–47%
Erythrocyte sedimentation rate:	0–20 mm/h	0–30 mm/h

	Male	Female	Newborn	Age 1
ALT:	10–52 U/liter	7–30 U/liter		
AST:	11–40 U/liter	9–26 U/liter	35–140 U/liter	20–60 U/liter
Creatinine:	0.8–1.5 mg/dl	0.6–1.2 mg/dl	Lower for children	
Creatinine kinase:	61–200 U/liter	30–125 U/liter		

Albumin:	3.5–5.0 gm/dl
Serum glucose (fasting):	65–110 mg/dl

Alkaline phosphatase:	39–117 U/liter
Total bilirubin:	0–1.2 mg/dl
Lactate dehydrogenase:	108–215 U/liter

CSF glucose:	50–75 mg/dl
CSF protein:	15–45 mg/dl (20–80 mg/dl)
CSF total nucleated cells:	0–3/mm^3

Body temperature:	37°C
Heart rate:	60–100/min; higher for infants and children
Respiratory rate:	9–18/min; higher for infants and children
Blood pressure:	90–150/50–90; lower for infants and children

LIST OF FIGURES

GLOSSARY OF MEDICAL TERMS

The purpose of this glossary is to define, in simple terms, medical terminology which may not be familiar to individuals using this book. It is not an exhaustive listing, and microbiologic terms are not defined. Access to a medical microbiology or infectious disease text will be required for determining the meaning of microbiologic terminology used in this text.

adenopathy: an enlargement of lymph nodes in response to some stimulus such as inflammation or infection; can occur singly or in multiple nodes.

agglutination: the interaction between a particulate antigen and antibodies specific for the particular antigen; the antigen-antibody complex leads to the aggregation or clumping of the antigen-containing material.

alveolus: an air sac in the lung consisting of a single layer of cells surrounded by a network of capillaries also consisting of a single cell layer; gas exchange occurs here.

anergy: a lack of the ability of the immune system to respond with a delayed type hypersensitivity reaction to commonly and previously encountered antigens such as mumps and candida; often seen in patients with AIDS.

annular rash: flat, ringlike lesions on the skin.

anorexia: decreased appetite.

antipyretics: fever-reducing agents such as aspirin, acetaminophen, or ibuprofen.

Apgar score: an assessment of a newborn infant using respiration, heart rate, muscle tone, reflexes, and color; usually done at 1 and 5 minutes after birth; a maximum of 2 points is determined for each category for a possible total of 10.

aplastic anemia: decrease in the numbers of all elements in the blood due to the death of their precursor cells in the bone marrow, where the cells usually mature; often associated with drugs which are toxic to these cells.

appendectomy: surgical removal of the appendix (vestigial part of the large intestine) usually because of acute inflammation.

arthritis: inflammation or infection of a joint, leading to decreased and painful mobility of the affected joint.

arthrocentesis: removal of synovial (joint) fluid through a small needle inserted in the joint cavity.

asplenia: absence of the spleen, either congenitally (at birth) or later, often seen in persons with long-standing sickling disease. This condition makes the individual susceptible to infections by certain bacteria.

auscultation: a method based on sounds or sound changes, used during a physical examination to gather data on internal organs like the heart, lungs, liver, etc.; the most common method involves the use of a stethoscope.

axillus: armpit; the area between the upper arm and chest wall where the two join.

bibasilar: pertaining to the bases of both lungs.

bilateral: pertaining to both sides of a symmetrically shaped tissue, organ, or the entire body; for example, the right and left lungs are bilateral organs.

biliary tree: system of ducts through which bile is transported.

bronchitis: inflammation or infection of the airways.

bronchoalveolar lavage: the instillation of saline fluid into the airways of the lungs so that samples can be removed and the washings (fluids) can be analyzed for malignancy or infection; also done during bronchoscopy.

bronchoscopy: the use of a flexible hollow tube to look directly at the trachea, bronchi, and larger airways in the lungs; it is also possible to obtain samples (biopsies) through this device.

bronchospasm: episodic constriction of smooth muscles lining the bronchi in response to some kind of irritant or stumulus.

buccal cellulitis: inflammation or infection of the cheek, often not well localized.

calcification: focal area of increased deposition of calcium compounds.

carbuncle: infection involving more than one hair follicle; usually seen as a merging of individual boils (furuncles) and often caused by *Staphylococcus aureus.*

CD4-positive cells: subset of T lymphocytes which are characterized by the presence of CD4 receptors on their cell membrane surfaces; they assist in turning the immune response on by activating other T and B lymphocytes. Also called T-helper cells.

cellulitis: inflammation or infection of tissues beneath the skin.

cerebellar: pertaining to the cerebellum (the portion of the brain concerning the coordination of complex movements and balance).

cerebrospinal fluid: fluid surrounding the brain and spinal cord.

cervical: pertaining to the neck or necklike portion of an organ.

chemoprophylaxis: the use of chemicals such as antibiotics to prevent the occurrence of disease.

cholangitis: inflammation or infection of the bile ducts.

chorioretinitis: inflammation or infection of the light-detecting layer (retina) and the underlying vascular tissue (choroid) beneath it in the back of the eye, which can lead to progressive impairment of vision.

cirrhosis: destruction of a tissue or organ with loss of normal structure which is replaced with scar tissue; common in association with alcoholism, where it involves the liver.

conjunctivitis: inflammation or infection of the tissue protecting the front of the eye.

coryza: acute inflammation or infection of the nasal membranes, leading to a thin watery discharge from the nose, as is seen with the common cold.

costovertebral angle: the area in the back where the last ribs join to their respective vertebrae.

cushingoid body habitus: an increase in adipose tissue (fat) in certain areas of the body, legs, and trunk. Purplish stripes, especially on the abdomen (striae), are also seen associated with Cushing's disease.

cystitis: inflammation or infection of the urinary bladder; also called a urinary tract infection (UTI). Associated with symptoms including painful urination, increased urination, and/or malodorous urine.

cytomegalic: pertaining to abnormally large cellular components, associated with infection by cytomegalovirus (CMV).

cytopathic: changes in intracellular structures due to disease or toxins, usually leading to the death of the cell.

dermatomal: pertaining to the area of skin which is served by one sensory spinal nerve.

desquamation: sloughing or peeling of the upper layers of the skin.

disequilibrium: unsteady balance.

disseminated intravascular coagulation (DIC): a phenomenon which arises due to the depletion of clotting elements in the blood, caused by many disease processes; diffuse, severe hemorrhaging can occur; without treatment, this is usually fatal.

dorsal: referring to the back or posterior aspect of a tissue or organ.

dorsal root ganglion: group of nerve cell bodies outside the spinal cord which convey sensory impulses to the brain.

dyspnea: difficulty breathing; also called shortness of breath.

eczema: an itchy, scaly, blistery or raised rash often seen in children and associated with irritation of the skin.

emphysema: abnormal trapping of air in the lungs due to loss of elasticity of the tissue, leading to a large, barrel-shaped chest because of the resulting overinflation of the lungs; also called chronic obstructive pulmonary disease or COPD. Often seen in smokers and in certain enzyme deficiencies.

empyema: the collection of purulent material in the pleural space.

encephalitis: inflammation of the brain.

endobronchial: pertaining to a location within a bronchus.

endocarditis: inflammation or infection of the tissue lining the inside of the heart; usually involves the heart valves.

endometritis: inflammation or infection of the lining of the uterus (womb).

endoscopy: procedure involving the passage of a flexible hollow tube into the esophagus and gastrointestinal tract, allowing its direct visualization; also useful for obtaining samples.

eosinophilia: increased number of eosinophils (type of leukocyte) in the blood, often associated with parasitic infections.

eosinophilic meningoencephalitis: infection of the brain and its coverings by parasites, leading to a vast increase in the number of eosinophils (subset of leukocytes) in cerebrospinal fluid or affected tissue.

epiglottitis: inflammation or infection of the flexible flap of tissue which covers the larynx during swallowing.

epilepsy: seizure disorder caused by abnormal electrical activity in the brain; may or may not be associated with motor movement, but the state of consciousness is almost always affected by the event.

epitrochlear: referring to the area of the upper arm just above the elbow, involving the bony projections (condyles) of the humerus nearest to the elbow joint.

erythema: reddening, usually of the skin or mucous membranes.

esophagitis: inflammation of the esophagus.

ethmoid sinus: air-filled cavity in the ethmoid bone located below the orbit of the eye and beside the nose.

extensor surface: the surface of a joint involved in extension or straightening of a limb.

extradermatomal: not confined to one dermatome.

extrahepatic: any place in the body outside the liver.

extramedullary cranial ganglion: outside the medulla oblongata (brain-stem), in reference to the cranial nerves.

exudate: fluid resulting from inflammation or infection; contains an increased number of cells and an increased amount of proteins and other cellular debris.

folliculitis: inflammation of hair follicles (place where the hair shaft penetrates the upper skin layers).

fontanelle: soft area between the cranial bones of an infant's skull, indicative of areas not yet ossified.

furuncle: a localized infection of one hair follicle and its surrounding tissues, usually caused by *Staphylococcus aureus;* also known as a boil.

gastritis: inflammation of the stomach, usually only involving the lining inside this organ.

granuloma: a collection of leukocytes, macrophages, and specialized cells of the reticuloendothelial system surrounding a focal area of chronic inflammation or infection; usually forms a nodular mass.

granulomatous: pertaining to or resembling a granuloma.

Guillain-Barré syndrome: inflammation of peripheral nerves leading to increasing weakness or paralysis; most often occurs in more distal areas before affecting portions of the body more proximally. Usually remits with the resolution of the underlying disease.

hematocrit: amount of red blood cells (erythrocytes) in a given volume of blood; usually expressed as a percentage.

hematuria: the presence of blood in the urine.

hemophilia: a bleeding disorder caused by a deficiency of clotting factors in the blood; occurs in males who carry the abnormal gene (on the X chromosome).

hemoptysis: coughing up (expectoration) of blood or blood-streaked sputum from the lungs.

hepatitis: inflammation of hepatic (liver) cells.

hepatosplenomegaly: enlargement of the liver and spleen.

horizontal transmission: passage of disease from person to person or by contact with infected materials.

humoral: referring to substances in the blood; in the immune system, this refers to antibodies to help fight disease rather than the cellular portion which involves leukocytes.

hypopituitary: pertaining to a decrease in the amount of hormones produced by the anterior (forward) portion of the pituitary gland; involves hormones which affect growth, steroid production, thyroid gland function, and the regulation of the female reproductive cycle.

hypotension: abnormally low blood pressure.

hypoxemia: low oxygen content in the blood.

idiopathic cardiomyopathy: dilatation and weakening of the heart muscle with no known cause.

impetigo: infection of previously damaged skin by group A streptococci or staphylococci; lesions usually drain honey-colored fluid.

induration: firmness in soft tissue.

infarct: tissue death often due to an interruption in the blood supply to that tissue.

infiltrate: the invasion of the spaces in a tissue by materials not usually found in the tissue, such as tumors, infectious agents, white blood cells, etc.

interstitial: spaces between the components of a tissue; e.g., in the lungs this pertains to spaces between the lung parenchyma.

intrauterine: inside the cavity of the womb, as for an unborn child.

in utero: inside the womb.

jaundice: yellow cast of the skin and mucous membranes due to an increase of bilirubins (bile breakdown products) which occur because the liver is unable to clear these chemicals from the blood; often due to toxic or infectious hepatitis.

keratoconjunctivitis: inflammation or infection of the outer covering of the eye, including the cornea.

ketoacidosis: a decrease in the pH of the body due to the accumulation of ketones in the blood and tissues; often seen in diabetics with poorly managed disease. Reverses with treatment and resolution of the underlying cause.

laparotomy: surgery to gain access to the abdominal cavity.

laryngitis: inflammation of the larynx (voice-box).

laryngotracheobronchitis: inflammation of the larynx (voice-box) and larger airways.

lethargy: drowsiness or decreased responsiveness.

leukocytosis: an increase in the number of white blood cells in response to some stimulus.

leukopenia: a decrease in the number of white blood cells.

lymphocytosis: increase in the number of lymphocytes above normal.

lymphoma: cancer of the lymph cells or their precursors.

lymphoproliferative disorders: any one of a group of cancers involving cells from which white blood cells or platelets are derived; includes lymphomas, leukemias, and multiple myeloma, among others.

macular: pertaining to lesions which are flat and which are often only detected because of a change in color or texture of the lesion from surrounding, normal tissue.

maculopapular: pertaining to lesions with properties which are both macular and papular.

malabsorptive diarrhea: an increase in the total number or volume of stools due to a decrease in the absorption of nutrients (especially fats) in the small intestine.

malaise: generalized feeling of discomfort caused by any disease process.

mastitis: inflammation of the breast.

meninges: thin, tough tissue surrounding the brain and spinal cord.

meningitis: inflammation of the meninges.
   aseptic: low number of white cells in cerebrospinal fluid, predominantly lymphocytes, most frequently caused by infection by viruses or fungi.
   septic: high number of white cells, predominantly neutrophils, due to infection by bacteria.

metastasis: the occurrence of disease at sites distant from and not connected directly with the site where the disease first appeared; this process is seen with many tumors and infections.

mitral regurgitation: any condition of the mitral valve between the left atrium and left ventricle that allows blood to flow back into the left atrium when the ventricle contracts; normally, the valve shuts tightly, allowing no flow of blood back into the atrium; often heard as a heart murmur during auscultation.

mitral valve prolapse: a defect of the valve between the left atrium and ventricle caused by a weakening of the tough, connective tissue of the valve leaflets, which allows the valve to project back into the left atrium; during normal operation, the valve closes tightly during ventricular contraction.

morbilliform rash: rash which resembles the flat to slightly raised (maculopapular) lesions seen in measles.

mucocutaneous: involving the skin and mucous membranes.

myalgia: soreness or aching of muscles.

myocarditis: inflammation of heart muscle cells.

nodular: knotlike or raised, solid lesions of the skin or other organs.

nonsuppurative sequelae: complications, caused by a previous attack of a disease, that do not contain or drain pus.

normotensive: normal blood pressure; the usual readings in adults are seen between 90/50 and 150/90.

nosocomial: any hospital-acquired condition resulting from a person's hospital stay.

nuchal rigidity: stiffness of the neck, often associated with meningeal infection.

occult blood: blood present in body fluids such as stool which cannot be detected with the naked eye; the most rapid test for occult blood is a guaiac (Hemoccult) test.

opisthotonic: spastic state in which the head and heels are bent backward and the torso extends outward.

opsonic: pertaining to an agent (typically an antibody) that, when bound to an antigen such as bacterial proteins, enhances the ingestion of the antigen by white blood cells.

orthostatic hypotension: decreased blood pressure caused by standing erect; often seen in patients who are dehydrated.

osteomyelitis: inflammation or infection of bone.

otitis media: inflammation of the middle ear behind the ear drum; visualized with an otoscope, which often shows the presence of fluid or pus behind the ear drum.

papular: pertaining to lesions which are raised and well circumscribed.

papulosquamous lesions: papular lesions which are scaly or peeling.

parasitemia: presence of parasites in the blood.

paresis: incomplete paralysis.

paroxysm: the abrupt episodic recurrence of disease or disease symptoms; also, spasms or fits.

pathognomonic: symptoms or lesions characteristic of a single disease process, on the basis of which a diagnosis can be determined.

pericarditis: inflammation of the sac covering the heart.

periorbital: around the eye socket (orbit).

periosteum: tough tissue surrounding the surface of any bone.

periumbilical: pertaining to the area surrounding the navel (umbilicus).

petechiae: pinpoint, flat lesions due to hemorrhage of blood into tissues under the skin or mucous membranes.

petechial rash: small, pinpoint, and flat lesions of the skin and mucous membranes associated with hemorrhage beneath the tissue; similar to purpura, except the lesions seen with purpura tend to be larger.

Peyer's patches: lymphatic tissues in the walls of the large intestine.

pharyngitis: inflammation of the pharynx, the muscular tube connecting the nose and mouth to the esophagus and larynx.

phenotypic: pertaining to the effects of an organism's genes and the environment on its physical appearance, biochemistry, and physiology.

photophobia: abnormal sensitivity to light.

pleurodynia: episodic pain due to transient intercostal muscle (muscles between the ribs which assist in respiration) spasms, caused by irritation of pleura.

pneumonia: infection of the lung parenchyma.

polyarteritis nodosa: inflammation of medium and small arteries, causing rashes, lesions, or organ damage to areas served by the affected vessels.

preeclampsia: a condition of the late stages of pregnancy caused by the accumulation of toxins in the blood; characterized by high blood pressure, swelling of the hands and feet, and the presence of proteins in the urine. If seizures are present, it becomes known as eclampsia.

preauricular: pertaining to a location just in front of the ear.

proctitis: inflammation of the rectum.

proctocolitis: inflammation of the colon (large intestine) and rectum.

prophylactic: pertaining to agents or procedures which prevent disease processes in susceptible individuals; for example, giving vaccines or antibiotics to prevent infection before it occurs.

prosthetic: pertaining to a man-made replacement for a missing or defective body part, such as artificial limbs or heart valves.

proximal phalanx: the part of a digit (fingers or toes) that is closest to its attachment to the body.

ptosis: drooping of the upper eyelid.

punctate: pertaining to lesions or markings which look like points or dots.

purpura: purplish lesions of the skin and mucous membranes due to hemorrhage beneath the tissues; usually less than 1 cm in size, lesions may be flat or raised.

pustular: pertaining to a skin rash with the presence of pus in the lesions.

pyelonephritis: infection of the kidney with or without a concurrent bladder infection.

pyuria: the presence of pus in the urine.

rales: abnormal breathing sounds heard by auscultation of the lungs during respiration; classified as dry or moist.

renal: pertaining to the kidney.

reticulendothelial system: the specialized white blood cells (especially macrophages) and other cells in the lymph nodes, liver, and spleen.

retinal: referring to the retina.

retinitis: inflammation of the light-detecting tissue (retina) in the back of the eye.

rhinitis: inflammatory or infectious process involving the mucous membranes lining the nose.

rhinorrhea: thin, watery discharge from the nose; runny nose.

rhonchi: coarse, low-pitched sounds associated with the presence of secretions or obstruction of larger airways in the lungs during inspiration and expiration.

ring-enhancing lesions: lesions in the brain seen on computed tomography (CT) scans, consisting of lucent (less dense to X rays), rounded masses surrounded by a region of increased density, especially with the use of vascular contrast material; often seen in certain infections of the brain.

salpingitis: inflammation or infection of a tube; usually the Fallopian tubes between the ovaries and the uterus.

scarlatiniform: pertaining to a skin rash resembling the red, coalescent (joining of many lesions), nonraised rash seen in scarlet fever.

septic abortion: infection of the mother after the abortion of a fetus; can involve the uterus and become a widespread systemic infection.

septic arthritis: painful, swollen, or stiff joints resulting from the presence of bacteria in the joint space.

septic embolus: clot (blood or other occlusive material) carried by the blood which contains infectious agents; often leads to systemic infection. Its occurrence can be sudden.

sinusitis: inflammation of the sinus cavities, often leading to headaches or nasal congestion.

splenomegaly: enlargement of the spleen.

spongiform: pertaining to a spongelike appearance; when this is noted in brain tissue, it is indicative of the presence of Creutzfeldt-Jakob disease or another slow virus disease.

stillbirth: birth of a nonviable infant, with death occurring at any time before birth.

stridorous cough: cough associated with laryngeal blockage which results in a characteristic high-pitched cough.

subcostal retractions: inward movement of the area between the ribs, associated with an increased respiratory effort.

superinfection: an infection by organisms because of a previously acquired, but ongoing infection (such as a bacterial pneumonia which sometimes occurs during or after a viral pneumonia).

suppurative lymphadenopathy: enlarged, tender lymph nodes from which pus is draining.

syncope: transient, brief episodic loss of consciousness (fainting).

tachycardia: increased heart rate (>100 beats/min in adults).

tachypnea: increase in respiratory rate (>20 breaths/min in adults).

tenosynovitis: inflammation of the tough sheaths surrounding tendons.

teratogenic: concerning agents which cause the abnormal development of an embryo, commonly resulting in fetal death or birth defects.

thrombocytopenia: a decrease in the numbers of platelets.

transbronchial biopsy: during bronchoscopy, the removal of a small piece of lung tissue through the walls of a bronchus (airway).

transplacental: crossing the placenta; pertaining to any substance which passes from the mother to the fetus or vice versa.

trismus: spasm of the jaw muscles.

tympanic membrane: the ear drum.

vaccine: the use of weakened (attenuated) or dead (inactivated) bacteria or virus, inactivated toxin (toxoid), or genetically engineered component of an infectious agent to promote immunity against a disease (such as smallpox or diphtheria).

vasculitis: inflammation of blood vessels leading to lesions on the skin, mucous membranes, or internal organs.

vertical transmission: passage of an infectious agent from the mother to an unborn child.

vesicular: pertaining to small, blisterlike lesions filled with clear fluid.

vesiculopustular: pertaining to blisterlike lesions containing pus.

zoonotic: pertaining to diseases or conditions usually affecting animals other than humans; however, following contact with infected animals or their tissues, humans can become infected.

INDEX OF KEY TERMS BY CASE†

† Numbers represent case numbers in the text.